G-STRINGS AND CURLS

By Tony Kaye

as told to Richard Seamon

Published 2007 by arima publishing

www.arimapublishing.com

ISBN 978-1-84549-180-2

© Tony Kaye & Richard Seamon 2007

Printed and bound in the United Kingdom

Typeset in Palatino Linotype 11/14

swirl is an imprint of arima Publishing

arima publishing
ASK House, Northgate Avenue
Bury St Edmunds, Suffolk IP32 6BB
t: (+44) 01284 700321

www.arimapublishing.com

Acknowledgements

Putting this together has been enjoyably hard work. The memory isn't what it was so I've had to resort to several parties to give it a jog or check that whatever I'd remembered, I'd remembered correctly. The British Library, as always, has been wonderful and I could have spent weeks in there. The Internet is a never ending source of information and the following sites and message boards have been no end of help, notably whirligig-tv.co.uk, simplonpc.co.uk for their unrivalled knowledge of ship names and service dates; cruise-critic.com and ssmaritime.com for background information on the Lakonia.

Also Lionel Titchener of the Tattoo Club of Great Britain for giving some ideas about my father's butterfly tattoo and Michael Hallinan, biographer of Bert Assirati and whose knowledge of wrestling is unparalleled.

Finally, I believe they call a person who writes on behalf of somebody else a ghostwriter. Richard Seamon, who made sense of my words is no ghostwriter. He had more patience than any man I've known, checked every story I told him and jogged my memory more than any psychoanalyst. It was hard work trying to recall events from over sixty years ago and so many times over the past year I was going to tell him I was going to give up. He must have been telepathic though. When I was at my wits' end I would sit down in front of the computer, open up an email from him and it would be about a musician I'd worked with sixty-three years ago and the memories, along with my enthusiasm, would come flooding back so banishing all the negative thoughts. Thank you, Richard. I'm amazed you stayed with me over the past year!

Anthony Kaye
London, October 2006

Preface

I've often been asked what I consider to be my biggest achievement or the most important thing I've done in my life. I've thought about this many times and come to the conclusion that apart from being blessed with a wonderful son, it has to be building a very successful business against all the odds after I was wrongly blamed for a tragedy. Although I don't actually see the end result as an achievement, I feel it was the successful culmination of all the things I've done throughout my life. Some tell me I'm lucky but I firmly believe in serendipity or being in the right place at the right time. I also believe strongly in destiny and I've always had that happy knack of being able to make the most of the opportunities that have sprung up for me, quite often out of the direst adversity. Each one of these events - and this is the thing that fascinates me to this day - has led on in one way or another to the next.

I've been lucky to have encountered a huge number of amazing people along this journey; from colourful East End villains through Hollywood stars to ruthless international businessmen. Some of these have been wonderful and generous, others have been thoroughly unpleasant but I have not written this book to settle scores or embarrass people because this has never been my way. If ever I've had an argument, I've had it in private and I do not wish to rake over the old ground of my personal or business lives here because this certainly isn't a "kiss and tell" story.

Finally, I've never kept a diary. These are memories pure and simple and as is the nature of memories, some are fresher than others and I'm sure we all understand that phenomenon. These are the ones I've managed to salvage and put in some form of order. I hope you enjoy them.

Chapter 1
Evacuated

It was late summer 1939 and the nation was on the cusp of war with Nazi Germany. To escape Hitler's impending bombs I, a scared little 12 year-old boy, along with the rest of my school, was evacuated from the heart of the East End of London to rural Fakenham in Norfolk. Little was I aware, as I stood waiting to be billeted, that I was forging the first link in the chain of events that would form the pattern for the rest of my life. Mrs Pointer, the woman who would be my so-called foster mother, was a complete tyrant and she could easily have got a job in a concentration camp. She scared the living daylights out of me right from the start.

That first night in her house was the first I'd ever spent away from home, so I was already nervous when this horrible and fierce woman showed me to my room and told me to go to bed. I didn't know where the toilet was and as I was too scared to ask, the inevitable happened and I peed the bed. Naturally I woke up horrified so I got up and tried to dry it but to no avail. I made the bed up again naïvely thinking that maybe it would be dry by the morning and that she wouldn't see it.

The next morning she marched me off to school alongside all the other evacuees. At 4 o'clock she came to fetch us home and I'll never forget what happened next. Grabbing me by my earlobe, she screamed that I was a "filthy disgusting tyke" then, still pulling me by my ear, marched me through the village to a doctor's surgery. As she yanked me into the consulting room she said to the doctor, "This disgusting creature wet the bed. Give him some pills to stop it immediately." That night I was so devastated I sent a letter to my parents saying that if they didn't come and get me, I would run away. I used to do everything I could to stay out of the house and away from the witch, including helping one of the other lodgers collect the eggs on the chicken farm he owned.

Eventually my father came up and took me back down to London. Had I stayed in Norfolk for the duration of the war, I'm certain my life wouldn't have followed the route it did. This one episode was almost a rite of passage in that it marked the end of my childhood and with my return to London, the end of my formal education. At 12 years old I was rudely inducted into adulthood.

Chapter 2
Gentlemen, We Work!

Home was 157 Osborne Road, Forest Gate, East London. The family had moved there from Hackney, where I had been born the younger of two brothers on the 21st August 1927, when I was four years old. When I was old enough, I attended Sandringham School in Sandringham Road but I was one of only a handful of Jewish kids there. There was a hell of a lot of anti-semitism about at the time and, being a bit of a natural fighter, as I got older and tougher I got myself involved in a few scrapes.

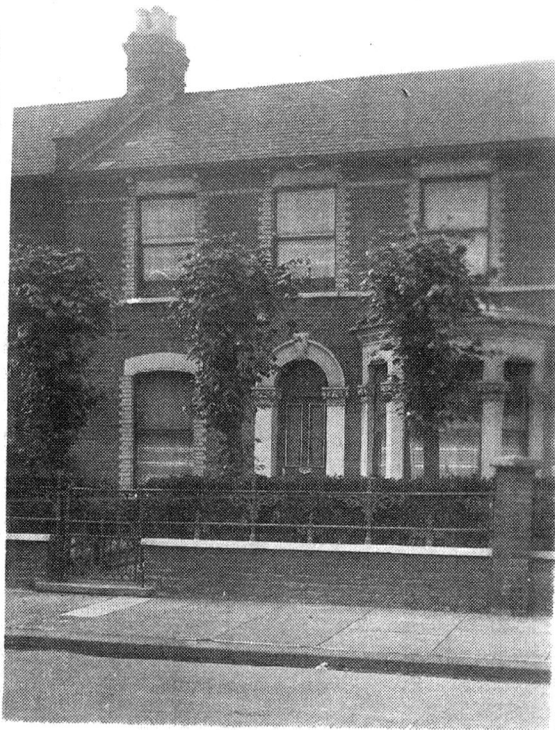

The family home, 157 Osborne Road, Forest Gate

I was about 11 years old when one day I came out into the playground to see all the kids ganging up on one poor boy and smacking him about. Fearlessly, I got in amongst them and pulled everyone apart. I knew who the ringleader was, a boy called Eric who lived in the next street from us and I went for him, kneeling on his shoulders and banging his head on the ground, letting him have a taste of his own medicine. Unfortunately I split his head open; not much, just enough for it to bleed and just enough to bring his parents into school the next day shouting the odds. They insisted I should be punished severely and even wanted me sent to Borstal for my actions. I can picture the headmaster's response, even today. He looked at them and told them bluntly:

"May I say that this never would have happened had you not been preaching anti-semitism in your home. Therefore, I'm not going to admonish Anthony. He'll be punished for his violence but that violence was provoked and I can understand how the five Jewish children in a school full of anti-semitism must feel."

He was a brave voice of reason at a time when feelings were running high in the East End following the Cable Street riots and other such events. Eric, seeing that I was handy enough to hold my own, stopped being a bully and wanted to become my friend. We ended up cycling out together, mainly speed racing. I'd tamed the beast; probably my earliest example of a talent for man-management!

I played cricket at school, too. I was the wicketkeeper for the school eleven and I was good enough to be noticed by Essex with a view to playing for one of their junior elevens. I was fearless and used to stand up to the fastest bowlers but I took lots of catches and made many a stumping because of it. It was to be my undoing though, as in one match I wasn't quite quick enough. I missed a ball and it hit me in the side of the face, knocking me out. When I came to I found that I didn't want to field close in and my sharpness had gone. I still love cricket though and my present house is just a few minutes from Lord's.

Although I'm Jewish, I have to admit that I'm not very observant. My parents used to uphold the high days like Yom Kippur and we'd light candles on Friday. My brother was Bar Mitzvahed but I wasn't because of the war getting in the way. And even though at one time father owned that most typical of Jewish establishments, a salt beef delicatessen, we certainly weren't very kosher as there was always plenty of bacon in the house for breakfast.

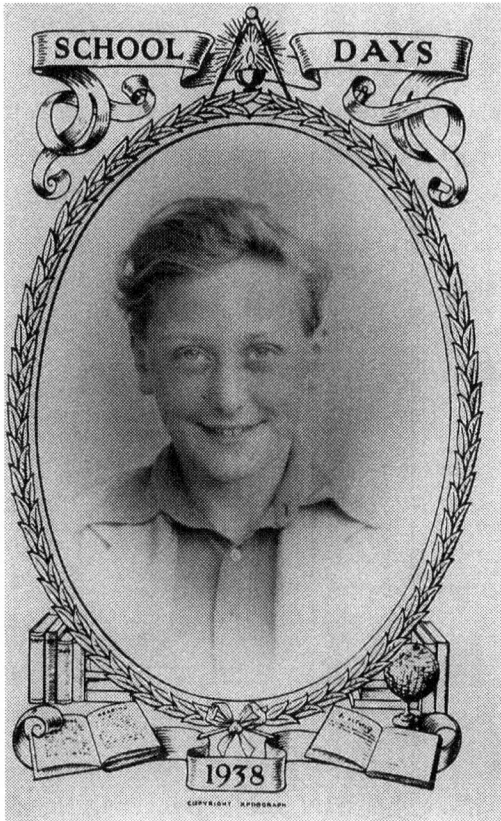

11 Years Old

My brother Bernard and I were born with the name Kaye but my paternal grandfather had fled from Poland to escape being conscripted into the army and his family name was Kronenburg. My father had anglicised his name to Kaye by deed poll to avoid the anti-semitism that was rife in the early part of the last century. Despite having little English my grandfather made some success of his life and ended up owning a lot of property. His father was apparently a baron and Grandfather had planned to go back to Poland to reclaim the property but unfortunately dropped dead of a heart attack one day while collecting his rents. Despite the intrigue, I've never been tempted to travel to Poland to check out the facts behind the story.

We were a pretty close extended family both geographically and socially. My mother's two sisters lived nearby, Aunt Polly and Uncle Mo opposite and Aunt Nan and Uncle Joe, two roads up in Windsor Road. Mo and Joe were also brothers who worked in the fish business. My brother and I were the only male children, as all my cousins were girls.

Every Tuesday and Thursday night we'd go across to Aunt Polly's and sit in the back room with a fire burning. Mother's brother, Lew, would be sitting there doing the crossword and the women would be gossiping. It was a very comfortable family scene. The only cloud over all this was my father. For reasons I've never understood he hated Aunt Nan and Uncle Joe so they could only visit us when my father wasn't there. It was sad but that was my father all over.

He had a terrible temper and he was the only blight on a perfect home life. One of my cousins used to beg my mother to leave him and even as an adult I used to ask her to come away with me. I hated him for the way he shouted at my mother and I can remember as a young boy beating my fists on his chest, calling him a dog and a pig because of it. I wouldn't have been surprised if mother had left him and I've long suspected that she may well have had a relationship with someone else but back then divorce was taboo, as well as being difficult to arrange, and many families just got on with it.

I'm certain that he suffered from what we now know to be obsessive compulsive disorders. Even the cat was terrified of him, haring downstairs from his illegal perch in the sun on hearing my father's approaching footsteps. Other occasions he would be shaving and would have to put his brush down several times until he was happy it was in the right place. This mania for arranging would even extend to people; we were both once stood in a queue at a bus stop and father was re-arranging everyone and yelling at them until they were the right distance apart. Of course now I realise that he was almost certainly ill but at the time he could be mystifying and often terrifying to be around.

The biggest influences you have as a child are your parents and that of my father, Sydney, was quite profound. He was an irrepressible opportunist; always with an eye for the main chance and sometimes those opportunities worked out. This was the more positive side of his character and thankfully this seems to be the part that rubbed off on me. Despite his problems, he was always interesting to be around, not least because there was always something going on.

There weren't many pies around without my father's fingers in them. He was an on-course bookmaker (he went by the name of Jack Lewis) and he also owned an amusement arcade in Deptford as well as the salt beef shop in Mare Street, Hackney. He worked the markets as well and sometimes I'd go with him. It was an education to say the least and some of the characters I was introduced to were larger than life.

It's fair to say that my father was to some extent a con-artist but then again, the areas he worked in were traditionally wide open for exploitation by those with an entrepreneurial streak or an eye for a quick killing and he was certainly gifted there. For instance, he had a guy working for him called "One-eyed Jack" who used to fix the one-armed bandits in the amusement arcade so they wouldn't pay out too much and there were other characters who hinted of an even darker element.

I was about eight or nine years old and we were at Romford market. A bowler-hatted man, whose face had more scar lines on it than Clapham Junction had railway lines, came up to us and started speaking to my father. His name turned out to be "Dodger" Mullins.

"Dodger," said my old man proudly. "I want you to meet my son. Dodger, show him the tools of your trade." And from his top pocket Dodger produced a pearl-handled cut-throat razor. I can still see the look on his face and I was genuinely terrified. He broke into a grin but it didn't take a genius to work out that Dodger's particular talent wasn't in a barbershop.

Father used to operate a well-known scam at the markets called the "run-out" or what would nowadays be called a mock auction. It was highly illegal but he took his chances.

I was with him once at Pitsea Market and he demonstrated to me how he could find out whether it was worth working or not, especially if there was somebody he recognised as a policeman about. This was called "getting the pitch in" and his method began with him throwing out cheap Japanese pens to everybody. By doing this he would start to draw a crowd around the stall.

When he saw the policeman move in he would pick up a rather more elegant pen and pencil set, a Swan with a gold nib or similar, but carry on dishing out the cheap ones.

"One for you, one for you, one for you and..." tossing the better pen toward the policeman, "One for you." And if the copper caught it, it was "Gentlemen, we work!" Then the real work would start.

It was a well-rehearsed and very effective scam. Members of the team planted in the crowd called "gees" would be scanning the rest of the crowd to see who had full wallets. If they spotted someone with some money they would signal my father who would then concentrate all his efforts into parting the poor victim from his money in exchange for a pile of cheap rubbish. It would invariably involve the gees coming in with fake bids and getting turned down in favour of the victim. By the time he realised he'd been done and wanted his money back, or - even worse - revenge, my father was long gone! Of course it was wrong yet it was crafty and convincing psychology and it was all sinking in to my young mind.

He was full of stories about how he tricked people. He especially liked to cheat the railways out of a fare. In the morning he'd carry an apple with him (this was back in the days when you only got apples in season) and as he passed through the ticket barrier he would say to the collector, "Good morning, George. How are you? I happened to be in the garden this morning, saw this apple and thought it would be ideal for you." Temporarily thrown by this unexpected act of generosity the collector would forget to clip my father's ticket.

When he was out working as a bookie, one of the clerks he had working for him was a tiny little guy called Bandy. Once while on the train coming back from the races they (father, Bandy and the other clerks and runners he worked with) heard the inspector coming along the train. They quickly put Bandy in the large bookmaker's satchel they had with them and slung it onto the luggage rack.

When the inspector came in they were all playing cards and when he asked to see their tickets my father asked him what he thought he ought to do with his hand. Obviously his reply wasn't all that generous and understandably he didn't give a damn about the hand, he just wanted to see the ticket otherwise he'd "Take that satchel and throw it out of the window." At which point a little voice came from the satchel, "Don't throw me out, Bandy's in here!" Exit one startled inspector!

But he could be a bitter man too and if he disliked someone it was forever. I witnessed this first hand at his father's funeral. Unable to forgive him for the death of his mother, my father, on being given the spade to turn the first soil back into the grave, threw both the soil and spade in together and shouting out after them, "Rot in hell, you bastard." It was an image I'd never forget; I didn't want to be like him.

In spite of my father's best efforts we weren't well off at all. If I ever saw my grandfather on the way to school I used to ask him if he could lend me a couple of pennies. Grandpa used to joke with me, asking me what security I could give him if he lent me tuppence. I used to offer my school cap and he would pat me on the head and send me on my way. Off I'd go to Barton's the Bakers and buy a penny worth of stale cakes from the day before, two doughnuts and two jam tarts – what a treat! The family was so poor they couldn't afford to pay for school lunch so I used to go to my aunt's house and have lunch with my cousins and while they feasted on chicken I, the poor relation, had to make do with sausages.

Father often lost all his money. Once, during the war, we were desperately poor and my mother asked her father to lend us £200. My mother was saying we'd soon be starving if we didn't get the money. Father went to my grandfather to collect it but was a long time returning. When he finally got back she asked him if he had the money with him. He said he had but when she asked him where it was he replied that he'd spent most of it already. Apparently there was a factory that had loads of flags and pennants left over from the coronation and he'd bought the lot for £180.

He reasoned that if we lost the war, as Jews we'd end up with nothing anyway and what money we had would be as worthless as toilet paper. On the other hand, if we won, everyone would want to wave a flag and want bunting and he'd be quids in. At the end of the war, the factory that originally sold it to him was the first to come back and ask to buy it back as, like most factories, their production had been turned over to the war effort and there was a shortage of available bunting. Unluckily for them, he'd already sold most of it on. I've always thought it was a stroke of genius and an indication of the great capacity for foresight he possessed and which I believed I inherited.

I'm still finding out things about him even now. Evidently he spent some time in prison for fraud when we were small children. I don't know quite when, where or for how long but I can remember he had a butterfly tattooed on his arm that he always tried to cover up whenever he wore a short sleeved shirt. Also he'd always dismiss our questions when we asked about it, as if it were taboo. I've since found out that this was a tattoo symbol commonly used in jail and associated with pickpockets. Somehow I don't think that was my father's style at all so it may well have just been symbolising his desire for freedom. Relatives have since told me that my mother used to tell my brother and I that he was away on business. I also came across a photograph of Bernard and myself from when I was about 4 or 5. On the back was a written message from my mother to father so I guess this must have been when he was inside. The strange thing is that while I must have been aware of it at the time, I have absolutely no recollection of him being away at all.

People have often said you can choose your friends but you can't choose your family. I think I was dealt cards off the bottom of the pack in that respect as my father was in such stark contrast to his brother, my Uncle Harry. They were like chalk and cheese, two completely different people. Harry was not only my favourite uncle he was a great friend and I always tried to spend as much time with him as possible.

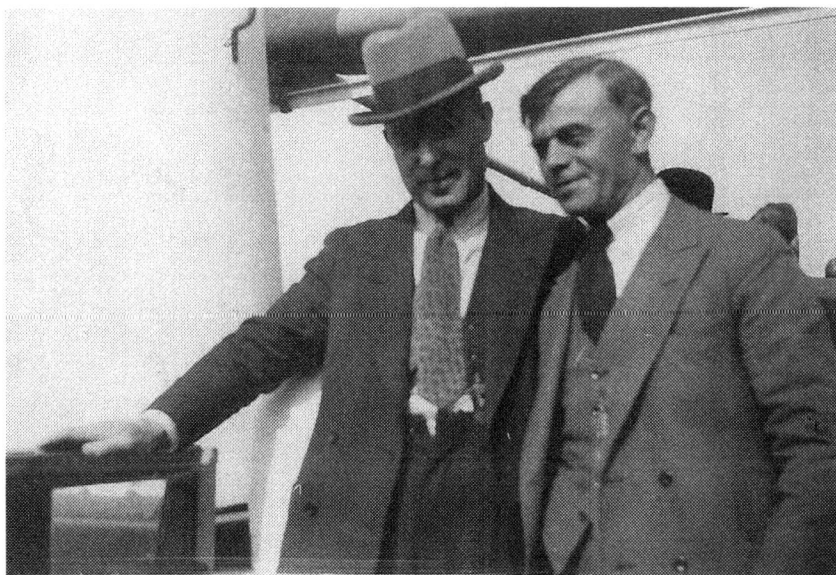

My father on the left and his fixer, One Eyed Jack

Chapter 3
Orchids and Gas Masks

So here I was at the beginning of a new life. My formal education was now over by dint of war and I had no qualifications. The only thing I'd been any good at in school was writing plays. They were performed though and I even won prizes – although they were usually only chocolate ones. I also remember my mother entering me for a musical competition or talent show when I was just 7 years old. When I walked on to the stage I apparently shouted out "Now it's my turn!" before I launched into my version of Shirley Temple's "At the Codfish Ball" which I rounded off with a tap dance. It was obvious there was a performer inside me just bursting to get out.

The bombing was getting worse and we were spending every night in the Anderson shelter at the bottom of the garden. It was freezing down there and all we had was a paraffin lamp to keep us warm. For entertainment, we used to take an old wind-up gramophone in with us and I can remember listening to the records of that great comedian Max Miller, "The Cheeky Chappie". I loved him and to this day I can still recite many of his songs and ditties. I think I probably developed my love of showbiz from him. Even though he was considered to be a bit risqué by the standards of those days, an uncle took me to see him at the Holborn Empire. I remember him coming on stage to his signature tune, "Mary from the Dairy" wearing his silk plus fours, his trademark Homburg hat and carrying a leg of ham.

"Guess What?" There were a few titters in the audience. "Queen Anne's." And off he went only to come back moments later with two bright pink potatoes. By now the audience was having convulsions. "You're all wrong, they're King Edward's" and down came the safety curtain. That, courtesy of the censor, was the end of the act. They were very strict back then.

Because of the relentless bombing, my father said my mother and I ought to get away out of danger so he arranged for us to stay with a couple in Hoddesdon in Hertfordshire.

While there I got a job in a garage. They taught me how to fix flat tyres and to change a wheel but they needed to see my insurance cards. As I was technically too young to be at work and really should have still been at school, I left before I was discovered. We then set up a stall in the local market selling cheap costume jewellery. On our first day there it was very foggy and all the jewellery started to go green! It definitely wasn't going our way so back we headed to London, preferring to take our chances among the bombs.

Despite my father being full of ideas it was actually one of my mother's schemes that helped to keep our family's heads above water throughout the war. When I returned to the East End from being evacuated there was no longer any school and it was the beginning of a new way of life for us all. There were also all these new things we had to do and learn about to prepare us for the inevitable hostilities. For instance, everyone had to carry their gas masks around all the time and I'm sure everyone's familiar with the cardboard box on string that they were kept in. Mother had the idea of making much more stylish cases, particularly for women.

Although we didn't have much money, Father was able to get hold of some rolls of cloth. He had some patterns made up and we set up a production line in the back room. Father drew the patterns out, my brother cut them out and Mother stitched them together. My job was to punch the holes out and put the press-studs in. Then it was everyone off to different markets to sell them.

They sold well but they also nearly got me killed. One day my Mother and I were on our way back from Gravesend market in Kent. We would cross the Thames on the ferry from Gravesend to Tilbury and catch the train back in to East Ham. This particular day also happened to be the one the Luftwaffe chose to bomb London for the first time. Earlier raids had been on industrial targets further down-river but this was the start of the blitz proper.

We got as far as Grays and the train was stopped because of bomb damage up ahead. We were evacuated from the train – all 500 of us – and into an unfinished air-raid shelter. Everyone was panicking because of the noise from the exploding bombs and the continuous ack-ack fire overhead. It was terrifying. Debris and shrapnel was flying onto the shelter and we didn't know whether to run for it or not. Those people trying to get into the shelter were all trying to squeeze through the small door together and it was pandemonium. This was new to nearly everyone after all and we'd not yet learned how not to panic. I don't know what prompted me to do it but I started to sing. Then everyone started to sing along with me and I ended up singing all night. We eventually got to East Ham station the next day where my father and Bernard, my brother, were waiting for us both fearing the worst. The local paper later printed a story about an "Unknown hero in the shelter" who started the community singing thereby stopping a lot panic induced casualties.

The only life I really knew anything of was the markets and I was becoming a bit of a wide-boy there, too. All that time I had spent with my father during the school holidays while he worked the markets had made me very streetwise and I wasn't afraid to say what I thought. I hatched a scheme to sell books from a stall and off I went to Watford market. I got the books directly from the publishers, Hutchinson, who happened to publish one of the biggest sellers of the day, "No Orchids for Miss Blandish" by James Hadley Chase, the British born writer of American style thrillers. However, me being me, I didn't just sell them, I came up with a better idea.

For instance, when a new Chase came out in hardback it retailed for 7/6d (37.5p). Realising that most of my potential customers couldn't afford that amount of money, I used to tell them that if they took really good care of the book, when they brought it back I'd give them half their money back. I found that with the war on, people were so concerned with economy they would go to great lengths to look after the books, often wrapping them in tissue paper or newspaper and that meant I would be able to sell them as new several times over. Not only that, I did the same thing with the second-hand books and I made a small fortune.

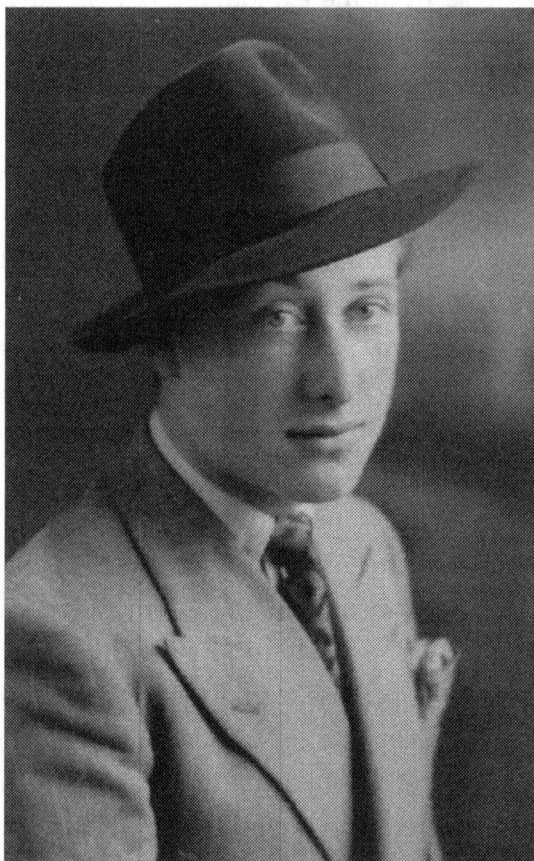

A Young Adult

However, selling books on the market wasn't always easy. One day a woman came along and asked who was selling "this disgusting literature" pointing towards the racy airbrushed cover of "No Orchids". I, being a typically cocky 14-year-old replied with a rather ill-advised "Piss off" and away she stormed. The forthright attitude

I'd inherited from my father was about to show me up as around an hour later a man in a raincoat and bowler hat turned up and began interrogating me.

"Are these your stalls?"

"Yes. And what the bloody hell's it got to do with you?"

"I'll tell you what it's got to do with me. I'm a police officer so you get that pornographic literature cleared up right away or you'll end up behind bars."

I telephoned Hutchinson's and they were very disturbed by the assertion that their book was pornographic. The cover may have been a bit suggestive, featuring as it did a girl wearing what appeared to be a see-through negligée but it certainly wasn't pornography. They were determined to fight and win a judgement and as I was a good customer of theirs they defended the case on my behalf. Unfortunately we lost as the market was on council property so they could effectively say what could and could not be sold with impunity.

Later on, the markets would be directly responsible for us getting our beloved Labrador dog, Peter. Peter was actually a bitch as we were unsure of her sex as a puppy so we named her after her previous owner, the very glamorous Lady Petrie. My father and brother had been selling furniture coverings from a stall in Colchester market and Lady Petrie was a regular customer, often bringing in eggs for them from her farm. Her pet labrador had had a litter of pups and she offered my father one. Peter turned into the most intelligent and lovable pet and I was immensely fond of her.

She would never go anywhere without a stick in her mouth. One day I went to take her for a walk but I couldn't find her stick anywhere. I used to smoke a pipe as a teenager so I grabbed a pipe out of the pipe-rack, put it across her mouth and off we went. Peter was happy as she had a stick and I never thought any more of it. We got down to the main road and were waiting to cross over. I noticed a lot of cars either slowing right down or stopping and looking at us. I looked down and amazingly Peter was sitting there with the stem of the pipe in her mouth in the conventional manner, looking for all the world as if she was enjoying a smoke! What's more, it was cold and the vapour she was breathing out looked like smoke. I took a picture of her dressed up and smoking the pipe and I still have it on display today.

She was a lovely docile dog but on one occasion a thief broke in through the kitchen window only to find Peter waiting for him and in no mood to welcome intruders onto her territory. She attacked him, biting his leg. As he made his escape the trail of blood he left behind helped to lead the police to him. Needless to say, Peter was one of the few good things to come from my father.

After the failure of the court case, mother said I ought to rent a shop and sell books legitimately. Father also tried to keep me in the markets by getting hold of some elastic for me to sell but when the supply ran out my thoughts turned elsewhere. Fate was going to play another hand – I was going to have a go at music!

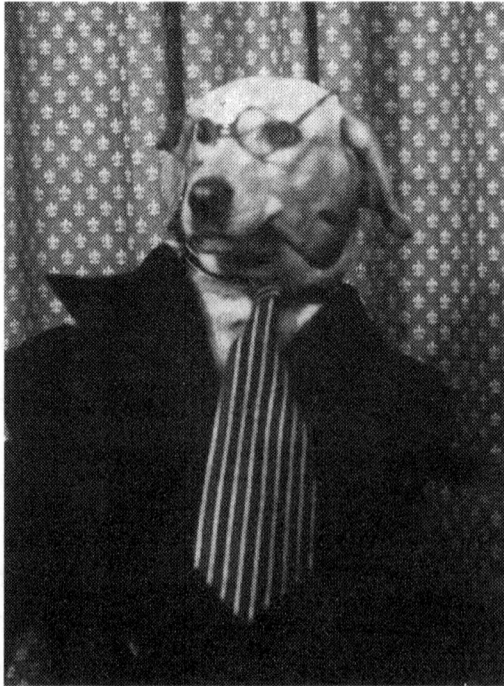

Peter

Chapter 4
I Got Rhythm

My interest in music came from my mother who, like many of her generation, played the piano. Not very well, I hasten to add but she played all the same. She always insisted that I took music lessons so I started with the piano and went on to the piano-accordion. I picked it up quite quickly and before long I could play a half-decent "Mexicali Rose". I wasn't brilliant but I was pretty determined. I just wanted to play music and I would even go to the Working Men's Clubs and play to the crowds there. I would do anything to just play and learn.

It was around this time that I began to get interested in jazz. I put this mainly down to my uncle Lew, the one who used to sit and do the crosswords by the fire at my aunt's. He used to bring along records by the likes of Duke Ellington and Louis Armstrong to play on the old wind-up gramophone and I was hooked. Bernard, my brother, bought a set of drumsticks and with him accompanying me on the biscuit tin drumkit, I used to try and play along to the records on the accordion! I loved it all and steadily became intoxicated by the likes Muggsy Spanier and Benny Goodman.

One day, in the back room of one of the clubs I saw a double bass. I looked at it, held it, messed around with it for a bit and without a clue about what I was letting myself in for, thought to myself that I liked this instrument and what's more, I liked it much more than I liked the accordion.

I took a trip to Ben Davis' Selmer musical instrument shop up the Charing Cross Road and there I found what seemed to be an old and decrepit looking double bass. I made a deal with them to swap my piano accordion for it. I was delighted - I was now the owner of a double bass! I was also the owner of a double bass and miles from home because I hadn't given a single thought as to how I was going to get this monster back from the West End to Forest Gate.

I struggled up to Tottenham Court Road and got on a 25B bus to Beacontree Heath. As I got on the conductor asked, "Where the bleedin' hell do you think you're going with that?" When I told him Forest Gate he said that as they were quiet, I could stand on the rear platform to Aldgate but that I'd have to change there. I managed to get on a Green Line Express bus at Aldgate, which was lucky because they had a big luggage platform. As soon as I got on I heard my first airing of a variation of the joke that has plagued double bassists for generations: "Oi!" yelled out the conductor, "I bet you can't get that under yer bleedin' chin!"

I got off the bus at Katherine Rd and I just happened to bump into my Uncle Mo, who ran a fish shop in Ilford market. He had a great sense of humour but he looked at me as if I'd just arrived from Mars as I struggled along, still trying to work out how to carry this immense instrument. "What the bloody hell have you got there?" he asked. He too followed his enquiry up with the inevitable "chin" joke. I must have heard it scores of times over the years and believe me, it doesn't get any funnier.

Now I had the instrument, all I needed to do now was learn how to play it. In those days there were theatres all over London. One of our local ones and the one we used to go to more often than not, was the Ilford Hippodrome. I went along there knowing that they had a pit orchestra so one day I went up to the bass player and asked if he gave lessons. He was a typical old-time musician with a beer-belly and as sarcastic as they come but he said he would teach me. I can't even remember his name or, for that matter whether I even knew it as everything seemed to be done on an anonymous basis.

As soon as he saw my bass at our first lesson he asked me where I'd bought it from. When I said I'd got it from Ben Davis he then asked me how much I'd paid for it. Then after I told him I'd traded in my accordion for it, he told me I'd actually got a very valuable instrument.

He said that it was originally a three string bass that had had an extra tuning peg added, so it was probably quite old. It was really only around the turn of the 20th century that double basses gained a fourth string.

I was an avid student and I learned everything I possibly could from him. After lessons, my brother Bernard and I used to go along to the East Ham Rhythm Club to listen to the musicians jamming. Among the players there were Tommy Callaghan on drums, Len Woods on tenor sax, Cecil Prestlin on alto and the great Bert Weedon on guitar. Bert's brother Mo played bass and I used to tell Bernard that I reckoned I was better than Mo even though I was only a novice, so he suggested I go and ask for a sit in. Eventually I plucked up the courage and they let me jam with them. They must have been impressed because they asked me to join them in their future sessions. It was unpaid but it was great experience. I found out later that they had had a good bass player but that he'd been called up into the RAF and Mo was just a reluctant stand-in.

It wasn't long either before I tried my hand at promoting. One of the local clubs was held in the basement of a dancing club run by an extremely gay chap called Herbert. He had a small ballroom with tables, chairs and also a kitchen. I asked him if he'd let me use it as a jazz club where on a Sunday afternoon people could dance and have a bite to eat. Surprisingly, he said yes. I got some of the musicians from the Rhythm Club together and formed a small band. I couldn't get a drummer so my brother Bernard, who messed around on the drums a bit, stood in. Not for long though as I remember that Herbert came to see our first session together. He took one look at Bernard and screeched at him to stop: "Stop playing trains! I can't bear it! You can't play bloody drums to save your life!"

I managed to find a decent drummer and the club became quite successful with many of the locals escaping the ravages and privations of war for a bit of light relief on a Sunday afternoon. Later, I was able to get guests to come down from the bands I was working with in the

West End; guys like Benny Lee who went on to sing with Johnny Claes and who also had quite a career both as a singer and as an actor.

My teacher was very honest and one day he said there was nothing else he could teach me and that if I wanted to have a career I ought to be smart and get to a college of music. I applied to the Guildhall School of Music and in May 1942 I was enrolled under the tutelage of Professor James Merrit, who also happened to be first bass with the BBC Symphony Orchestra.

I wanted more than anything to play jazz so my reasons for attending the school were quite selfish: I needed more knowledge of the instrument and to learn good technique so there was obviously going to be a little friction with my tutor's more classical outlook. My idol was the great Jimmy Blanton who played with Duke Ellington for two years from 1939 until TB forced his early retirement in 1941 and subsequently caused his early death a year later. Jimmy Blanton was a brilliant player who could make a double bass sound almost like a cello and I almost wore out my copy of "Pitter Panther Patter" trying to copy it. Legend has it that after his death, Blanton bequeathed his Panormo bass to the Ellington orchestra, to be used by whichever player stepped into his shoes.

Professor Merrit knew of my love for Jimmy Blanton and one day he told me that that very evening he, Merrit himself, was going to be playing in a wireless broadcast with Monia Liter and his 20th Century Serenaders. What's more, he was to be featured playing on one of my favourite Jimmy Blanton numbers, "Sophisticated Lady". He told me he wanted me to listen to the broadcast and he would discuss his performance with me the next day. I duly tuned in that evening.

"Well, Kaye," he asked at our next lesson. "What did you think?"

Dangerously I ventured, "Mr Merrit, technically you were brilliant but you have no soul, Sir."

"What do you mean, no soul?"

"When you play jazz, Sir, you need to play it from the heart and not from the brain; that's what makes wonderful jazz. You play what you feel. You were playing as if you were just reading the notes."

I can remember him standing there, looking out the window with an old Dragonetti bow behind his back, presumably letting my impudence sink in. Suddenly he whirled round, slapped me across the knuckles with the bow, told me I wasn't fingering correctly and to get on with my practice. I'm wondering now whether this episode had any bearing on his own career because I've since seen him cited as a respected jazz player and influence in his own right. Perhaps we were good for each other! At the time though, I began to think that this was going to be a competition on the rights and wrongs of jazz.

I was having trouble meeting the costs of the school fees. My parents had supported me at first because of the help I'd given them with the gas mask covers but now money was starting to get a bit tight. Then I landed my first job at the Granville Theatre in Walham Green, Fulham. It's no longer there having been controversially demolished in the very early '70s but back in the '40s it was still a grand old building by the master of Victorian theatre design, Frank Matcham. It even had the original gas lighting in the corridors. My debut didn't last long though because as soon as the curtain came up and we started playing, in marched some Military Police. They came straight onto the stage where they arrested the bandleader for desertion. The audience thought it was hilarious and all part of the act. We didn't though as it meant we weren't going to get paid. Instead we looked around to see what we could salvage from the mess in lieu of wages and I ended up with the bandleader's white tux - I thought I was cock o' the walk!

I'd heard from the guys at the Rhythm Club that Archer Street in Soho, just north of Shaftsbury Avenue, was the place jazz musicians socialised. The guitarist from the Walham Green gig, a guy named Laurie Deniz, confirmed this and said he'd meet me there the next Monday (Monday was always THE day for Archer Street) and introduce me to some of the guys. Laurie was the younger brother of legendary guitarists Joe and Frank Deniz and is the only musician I remember from that first gig, which shows what an inauspicious start to my professional career it was. Anyway, why not try it, I thought. I'd just about given up with the Guildhall by now because of the differences with Professor Merrit and not only was the desire to get out and play jazz overwhelming, so was the need to earn some money.

Incidentally, Joe and Frank Deniz lived long and productive lives. I recall going on a date to see the London production of the South African based dance musical, Ipi Tombi in the early '80s and as I walked into the theatre foyer I heard some quite wonderful live guitar music. I saw it was Joe playing but by now he was looking quite an old man. I went over to speak to him and he recognised me so we started talking about old times. Unfortunately I completely forgot about my date and never got to see the show but the reminiscing was wonderful!

I remember that first day at Archer Street very well indeed. The place was thronged with musicians because as well as all the agents' offices, the Musicians Union had their offices there. I met so many new faces as a result and felt that I'd become a bit more part of "the scene". Drummer Tony Crombie and saxophonist Ronnie Scott, long before he opened his famous Frith Street club, spring readily to mind as being about on that first visit. It was definitely a rewarding day too; I got a job and I was off to the seaside!

Chapter 5
Dance Hall Days

This was my first trip away from home since my evacuation to Norfolk but this one would hold happier and rather more exciting memories. The Brighton gig was with a band led by the redoubtable Ann Shar at one Brighton's major dance halls, Sherry's in West Street, which was then run by Mecca. She was a multi-instrumentalist but was very good at playing popular tangos for the dancers on the violin. Although well known, Sherry's had garnered a bit of a reputation between the wars as a bit of a rough-house and even got a mention in Graham Greene's novel "Brighton Rock".

Wartime obviously hadn't changed the atmosphere much. One of the regiments billeted to the area was the Canadian Black Watch and they treated the place like the wild-west or a gold rush frontier town. Every night the military police would arrive with whistles blowing and guns drawn as punch-ups flared and people were thrown from the balcony. It was like being in a Texas roadhouse with the band playing on as chaos reigned all around!

Sherry's was also where I got my first introduction to sex. There was a girl there who always seemed to be smiling at me while she was dancing. The drummer, a typically dour Scot, reckoned she fancied me and that I was on a dead cert. One day she came over to me and we got talking. She asked me where I was staying and I told her I had rented a bedsit in Hove.

"Why don't you let me go there and make tea for you for when you finish your afternoon session?"

That wasn't an offer I could easily turn down, even though I was still only 15. So, to cut to the chase, I finished work and went home.

We had tea and then we had some "afters" and I thought there and then that this musician's life was very definitely a great one!

That illusion was almost immediately shattered as I was startled awake by a loud banging on the door. I'd been lying on the bed half-asleep, very happy but also aware that I would soon have to get ready for the evening session. I opened the door and standing there was a guy in RAF uniform. There was no introduction and no further formality observed as BOSH! he hit me so hard that he sent me right across the room. My head hit the fireplace and I crumpled to the floor, stunned. All I could see now was this big pair of shiny boots making their way across the floor towards me when suddenly the door opened and in rushed the hitherto dour Scots drummer who luckily just happened to be staying next door and who'd heard all the commotion. He managed to wallop the airman just as I was about to get my ribs kicked in. I still had to turn up to work that evening with a swollen eye and lip.

Later that same evening, the airman actually came over to me and apologised. He told me that the girl was his ex-wife and that he was still in love with her. He was furious at what she had been up to since their divorce and his temper and jealousy had got the better of him. It was a rude introduction to the pleasures of the opposite sex but I'm pleased to say it never put me off them.

The Sherry's job came to an end after about 6 months and I headed off back to London. Now I knew what to do in order to find work quickly so the first available Monday I went up to Archer Street to find out what the gossip was and what work was about.

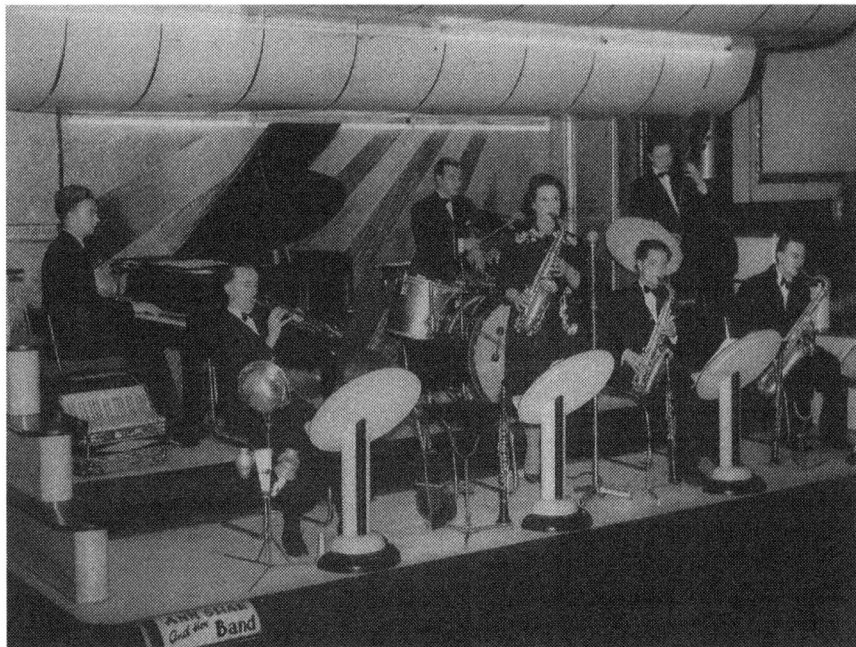

The Ann Shar Band. My rescuer on the drums to my right

I found out that the Panama Club in Knightsbridge was auditioning for bands to take over from the Johnny Claes Band. It was almost certainly due to the call up but there seemed to be a great shortage of bass players (did bass players make better soldiers?) and I managed to get auditions with half-a-dozen different bands, I was that determined. Harry Adams, the club's owner, told me after the final audition that I was sure of a gig as I was the only musician who'd tried out in every band! I actually got the job with the band led by trumpeter Dennis Rose. I needed a smart tuxedo as well so one of my uncles said I could borrow his. Trouble was, I was only around 15 so it was twice my size and I had to pull everything in with safety pins. One night I was playing and an uncle on my father's side, who was a bit of a playboy, came in and saw me.

"What the bloody hell are you doing playing here?" He politely enquired. "You should be at school!"

Well, being 15 or 16 years old at the time I didn't actually need to be at school because the leaving age was 14 back then but I told him to quieten down as the club would be closed if they knew I was under age. I said it was quite correctly illegal to employ children in nightclubs but I also told him there was a shortage of musicians and I was taking advantage of it before I got the call up to go and fight.

I played in many clubs over the next few years and often the work schedule was hectic. For instance, at one stage I was working with the Francisco Conde Band at Bentalls in Kingston for the afternoon dances and then I'd have to shoot back to the West End for the other clubs. Incidentally, Francisco Conde's real name was Franz Cohen and his band featured Eddie Calvert on trumpet, Malcolm Mitchell on guitar and Santiago Lopez on vocals, all of whom would go on to great things away from the band.

I have great memories of playing in the clubs over the next five years or so but while the memories are fresh, the advancing years have played merry hell with the filing system and getting it into any kind of order has been a nightmare! I've given up trying to work it out and even tapping the memories of the few surviving colleagues from that era hasn't yielded much as I fear we're all in the same boat. I was very young of course so many of my older contemporaries have long since departed, which is a shame but sadly inevitable. The internet though has been a great source of information and while it hasn't helped too much with the order, it has prompted many recollections to flood back.

The Panama was what we used to call a "Day Club" in that it ran from 8pm until midnight. At midnight the night was still young and many clubs used to go on until 4am, even during wartime, so as soon as the Panama had finished many of the musicians would pack up and dash off to the later-opening venues.

I'd secured a gig at the Astor Club in Park Lane; in fact I had two at the same time there. One of those was with someone who would become one of our greatest jazz pianists (finally honoured with an overdue knighthood in 2007), who was already making a name for himself, George Shearing and his quintet. The other was, once again, playing latin with Francisco Conde. The evening (morning!) was nonstop hour-long rotations with hardly a pause to breathe. Franz, or rather Francisco, would be playing a song at the changeover and lift off with his right hand. George would then slide in next to him to take up the melody with his right and off he'd motor. Brilliant, considering his blindness. It was the same for the other band members and I just about had time while all that was going on to slip out of my latin bolero jacket and change into a tux!

I had a natural talent for the bass and what I'd missed learning at the Guildhall I was picking up as I moved around from job to job. I found I could also emulate other players I'd heard on record pretty well. One of these was Slam Stewart who used to play "arco" (with a bow) and simultaneously hum an octave apart. This "unison" sound was very exciting and made the bass sound like a front line instrument. Most of all I was getting respect from my peers and it was a truly great feeling that I could hold my own musically with all these terrific players. It was a tough schedule but they were happy days and nights and I was enjoying every minute of it, whether I was playing jazz or big-band, sight-reading or improvising. Hard to believe I was still only a teenager.

Chapter 6
In the Clubs

Once again the Archer Street network went into action as Dennis Rose announced that he was leaving the Panama Club to front up his own band at the Jamboree Club in Wardour Street. There was a job there for me if I wanted it and I jumped in. The Jamboree was rather less formal than the Astor was and there were some splendidly eccentric goings-on, especially as there was also a striptease act in the cabaret.

I was playing so much by now that my young fingers suffered a lot. I tried everything going to try and harden them up but nothing would work. In the end I decided that every time I got a blister I would deliberately burst it and play on the new skin. It hurt like hell and I suppose I was dead lucky not pick up an infection but the fingers gradually became as strong as iron and they were fine.

The show featured a stripper, a girl called Pamela and she was the girlfriend of the owner, Bob Rowley. She used to do her act as we played "Taboo". After a while it actually became a bit of a pain in the neck having to look at her backside every night, but one particular evening was a bit different. There was always a bit of rowdiness but this night there was an American captain sitting at one of the ringside tables, becoming more drunk as the show wore on. Just as Pamela was about to get down to her g-string, the officer stood up.

"Godamm! I can't take it anymore, I gotta take a leak!" He yelled.

At which point he whipped out his John Thomas and peed on the floor. Some of it splashed up onto Pamela but Bob was like greased lightning, I don't think I've seen a man move so quickly! He went over to the American, grabbed hold of him, knocked him spark out then had him thrown out onto the street. A bouncer told me later that he'd been propped up in a doorway to sober up, well away from the club.

Another night, the Irish ex-boxer Jack Doyle was in. A decade earlier he was a household name and was said to have earned over a quarter of a million pounds from fighting, which was a huge amount in the 40s. Now he was sadly way past his best and he'd drunk and philandered away most of his fortune. This particular evening he was performing to type and was accompanied by a very pretty girl. As we were playing and everyone else was either drinking, talking or eating, we became aware of a man crawling along on his hands and knees. We were beginning to wonder what he doing when he crawled up behind Jack and cracked a bottle over his head. Jack must have had an iron skull because he just shook his head, turned round, picked the guy up off the floor and without much decorum, asked him what he was doing. It turned out that Doyle had been seeing his wife and that naturally this had upset him. Sadly for the poor cuckold, and as was normal with any troublemaker - regardless of whether he had a good excuse or not - he was thrown out.

The bandleader, Dennis Rose, was a great musician but it has to be said, a little on the weedy side, almost like a stick with very deep-set eyes. However, he wasn't without a certain amount of bravado. One night a Canadian officer complained that the trumpet Dennis was playing was a touch too loud and would he mind using a mute. No musician likes to be told how to play so Dennis responded by blowing even harder, this time right in his ear. Understandably upset, the officer responded:

"Goddammyou! I'm going to stuff this trumpet right up your ass!" and yanked Dennis off the bandstand. A mad panic ensued as the soldier was summarily ejected amidst visions of Dennis walking around with his trumpet rammed up his backside!

The relief pianist there was a guy called Barry Milne. He used to play with a glass of whisky at one end of the piano and a glass of gin at the other and was permanently as drunk as a lord. He did though have the most amazing musical brain. He could remember complete symphonies and play them back perfectly. You could name him a tune and he'd play it and even the famous conductor, Sir Malcolm Sargent, couldn't catch him out. He was a lovely guy and wouldn't harm a fly yet you could put him at a piano and he'd play wonderfully all day.

The marvellous thing about the Jamboree club was the after hours atmosphere. Musicians from all over would congregate there after their own gigs had finished for a jam and, from being a small band, we temporarily became a big one. The young Johnny Dankworth (now Sir John – our first jazz knight) and the Deniz brothers, Joey and Frank regularly attended the sessions and afterwards from about 4am onwards we'd head off to the Lyons Corner House in Coventry Street for breakfast. This was another great meeting place, always lively and full of fun as it would be thronged with all sorts of night workers such as ourselves and the local hookers. You took your fun where you could find it as the ever-present air raids meant every night could be your last gig. It was at the Corner House that I first encountered George Shearing's legendary (and revolting) breakfast combination of porridge and pickles. Quite how George managed it, I don't know but I've never forgotten it! 40 years later the memory of it would even come in quite handy.

I think it was also around this time that myself, Malcolm Mitchell on guitar and a friend called Barney Stockley on piano had a go on Carroll Levis' popular "Discovery Show", a radio talent show not unlike Opportunity Knocks. We appeared as the Malcolm Mitchell Trio and did it largely as a prank. Needless to say, we didn't win! Malcolm went on to become a very respected guitarist so we couldn't have been that bad.

It was during one of these jam sessions that John Dankworth told me that his bandleader at the time, Oscar Rabin, was looking for another bassist and that I should go and audition. The audition was at the Hackney Empire and unusually for me, I was very nervous. So if I was ever to mess up an audition it was going to be that one. The audition was set for the morning, which couldn't have been a worse time. I'd finished work at 4am then had to take the night bus back to

Forest Gate to get out of my tux so I just about made it to the theatre in time, although I was thoroughly exhausted. I was also beginning to wonder why I was there. The arrangement I was meant to play called for some arco and when I went to take the bow it fell out of my hand. I was angry with myself yet the cocky teenager took over and I gently put the bass down, said I didn't want to play arrangements or go on tour and walked out. As the bass wasn't mine and therefore unfamiliar, I was able to do this with some dignity. No more big bands for me, I thought, I'll stay with the little ones.

I went up to Archer Street and met up with Tommy, Len and Cecil, the guys from the East Ham Rhythm Club. They were all working with the Teddy Foster Band and, would you believe it, they needed a bass player! I thought it would be great to work with the guys from the club and I was buggered if I was going to be defeatist after messing up the Rabin try-out so I went up for the audition, met Teddy and got the job. So much for "no more big bands!" Because of a dropped bow, the Archer Street network had triumphed again.

Chapter 7
Teddy's Boy

Ironically, given that I'd just turned down a chance to go on tour with a big band and also play arrangements, I now seemed to be letting myself in for more of the same. It proved to be nothing of the sort and my time touring with Teddy Foster was just as enjoyable and eventful as the West End clubs. Teddy was on the Mecca dancehall circuit and we were off to play at the Corporation Street Mecca in Birmingham as our first call.

We were there for a time and got to know a few of the regular punters and, being a typical hot-blooded young male, I noticed one girl in particular. She was incredibly popular, especially amongst the lads, largely because she possessed the most tremendous chest. We all used to go into a pub following the afternoon session and on this particular day I'd been to the bar as it was my turn to buy a round. Unaware that the well-upholstered girl was standing right behind me, I turned round with an armful of drinks and my elbow hit her in the chest. She screamed and ran off to the toilet. I couldn't believe the pain I was in either as I thought I'd broken my arm. Later, when I looked at my elbow, I saw it was bruised black and blue. Even worse, I'd had to buy another round!

The girl turned up for the evening session but strangely her boobs didn't. My curiosity was getting the better of me so I went across and asked her why her boobs had almost broken my arm that afternoon. She explained that she'd been wearing falsies but because of the wartime shortages you couldn't get rubber ones anywhere and as she was a nurse, she'd used the plaster of Paris they made the plaster casts out of to make a set. She'd had to take them out because when I knocked into her, I'd smashed one!

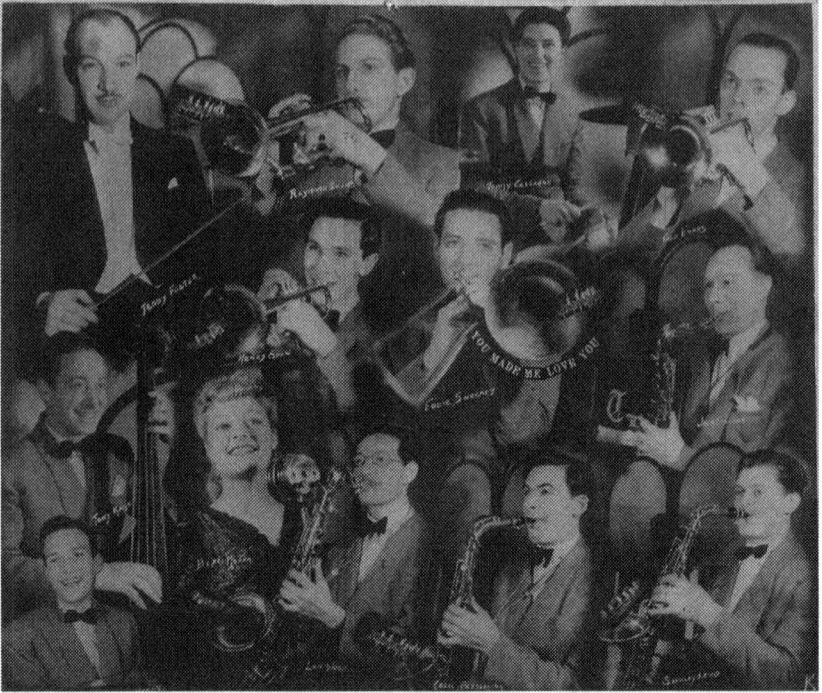

Taken at Casino Ballroom, Birmingham 1943.
Top:Teddy Foster, Ray Davies, Tommy Callaghan, Fred Evans.
Middle: Hank Shaw, Eddie Sweeney, Jack Collins
Bottom:Me, Alan Moran, Bebe Moran, Len Wood, Cecil Pressling, Stanley Lewis

One evening while in Birmingham I was visited after a show by our family doctor, who just happened to be in the city at a convention. I've never been sure why, but he always used to look upon me as his godson and that evening he introduced me to his colleagues as such. My mother was always very fond of him and although I've never been able to prove my suspicions, I've always felt that maybe he was able to give her some of the happiness she was missing from her marriage with my father.

After a while I'd had enough of Birmingham so I left the band and went back to London to play in the clubs again. Teddy came back and found me and asked me to rejoin the band for a variety show featuring the popular stand-up comedian Scott Sanders. So I went back but I was lucky to get out alive!

The second half of the show called for us to act as a turn of the century military band and we all wore moustaches (false ones if necessary) and pill-box hats with chinstraps in order to look the part. It was also meant to appear as if we were playing in a park. The stage was built up in a series of risers or rostrums and the top one held the drums, piano and myself on bass. Except that I didn't have a rostrum; I had a plank of wood with my bass at one end and a music stand at the other. Teddy came on as bandmaster and as the curtain went up he brought us all in on the down beat. As I hit my first note, my music stand went woosh, straight up into the gods and I crashed down onto the stage. Needless to say, the audience thought it was hilarious whereas I thought I'd broken my back.

"Don't just fucking lay there," spat Teddy from the side of his mouth, "play!" And he carried on conducting as if nothing had happened. Not that I could even if I'd been able to as my bass was split in half. That was during the matinee and the stage manager came on afterwards saying it was great and could we keep it in for the evening show?

After the variety show we went back out on tour. Very early one morning we arrived in a small village. We were tired and very hungry but it was so early that everything was still closed. The four trumpets had a great idea; they all got out into the middle of the village square and blew the Harry James arrangement - one that begins with an exceedingly rousing fanfare - of "Trumpet Blues and Cantabile". Suddenly all the lights came on and doors opened, revealing bewildered villagers who probably thought it was either the invasion or the King arriving. We just stood there looking sorry for ourselves and saying we were hungry. Luckily the locals were OK with us and we got fed; and as we were out in the country amidst plenty of farms, we got fed with loads of eggs and bacon and it was lovely! I can't remember the trumpeters' names who took part in that little stunt but two of my contemporaries during my time with the band were Ray Davies, later of "Button Down Brass" fame, and also the great Hank Shaw. Ray has since assured me that he wasn't there as he'd already left the band to get married but if one of them was Hank then the villagers were honoured!

Now my favourite uncle, my father's brother Harry, wore a ring that I really loved and secretly coveted. He'd told me a while earlier that when I made my first broadcast, it would be mine and it just so happened that the Preston show on our tour was going to be broadcast by the BBC. I phoned Harry up and told him to tune in because I was going to be on the wireless. We went on, did the show and then headed off back south to London. When I saw Harry I asked him for the ring. He was reluctant to part with it.

He told me, "I don't know if I should bloody well give it to you as you'd only been on for 10 seconds when the air raid siren went off and the radio was shut down." All anybody listening to the radio had heard of my first big band broadcast were the first few bars of our signature tune, "You Make Me Love You".

I would feature in a few more broadcasts though as dance band music was incredibly popular and morale boosting during those dark wartime days. One broadcast I certainly recall doing featured one of the great characters from that time, the trombonist Rube Stoloff, who used to follow the band around and probably deserves a chapter all to himself. He had played with the original Johnny Claes' Clae Pigeons but was now a member of the Billy Cotton Band. This particular broadcast was being done from the BBC Studios at the Aeolian Hall in Bond Street and we were installed nice and early for a 7am rehearsal.

During the rehearsal the sound man in the control room was complaining that I was too overpowering and that he couldn't get a good level on me. Eventually they put me in a corner with my back to the band but this meant I had to keep twisting my head round to watch Teddy conducting. By the end of the broadcast my neck was in agony and my throat was killing me as it had dried up with the strain of craning round all the time. I'd noticed that Rube had an atomiser spray that whenever we stopped playing he used to spray his throat with. Understandable; after all he was he was a blower and probably needed to lubricate every now and again. Or so I thought. He claimed that it had also been prescribed by his doctor for medicinal purposes and as such was personal and ought not be used by anyone else. Didn't matter to me, I grabbed it when he rested it on my music stand, saying that I needed something to relieve my dreadful sore throat. When I squirted it into my mouth I nearly choked – it was neat scotch! I should have realised as we all knew Rube was an alcoholic.

Another occasion at Covent Garden and Teddy wanted to introduce some choreography. The trombones were in front of the trumpets and he wanted them to swing in opposite directions as this would produce a great visual effect. Rube was so drunk that as the trombones swung one way, he swung the other but with just as much gusto and rather less control, right off the end of the podium and onto his back amongst the dancers. He just looked up at Teddy and said: "We didn't rehearse that."

He was a great joker though; in those days tuxedo shirts had collar studs and I always used to have terrible trouble fixing them, nearly always dropping them onto the floor. Whenever this happened, Rube would burst into a song and dance:

> "Silly old Tony, Silly old Tony,
> Gone and lost his collar stud,
> The silly cunt, I knew he would"

Then he would end his little dance with a jump and as he landed there would be a crunch – my collar stud!

Towards the end of the war we shared a slot at the Covent Garden Opera House, which had been converted to a dance hall, with Blanche Coleman's all-girl band. We'd do two shows a day, playing to 3000 in the afternoon then another 3000 in the evening and we had a huge amount of fun there. On VE Day there were thousands queuing up to get in and the buskers were working the crowd. In my infinite wisdom I reckoned this would be a great thing to do too, so I got some of the other guys from the band to join in, told the buskers to stop and to go round with the hat for tips instead. We started to play and everyone started dancing. The whole area in front of the Opera House boiled with people jitterbugging and jiving and even some police officers came out from Bow Street nick and joined in! Teddy wasn't quite so impressed though and he ended the festivities with a harsh, "What the fuck are you doing? I'm not paying you to play in the street."

So we packed up and went back inside. As we did so, I remember a busker coming up to me and thanking us because he'd never earned so much money before!

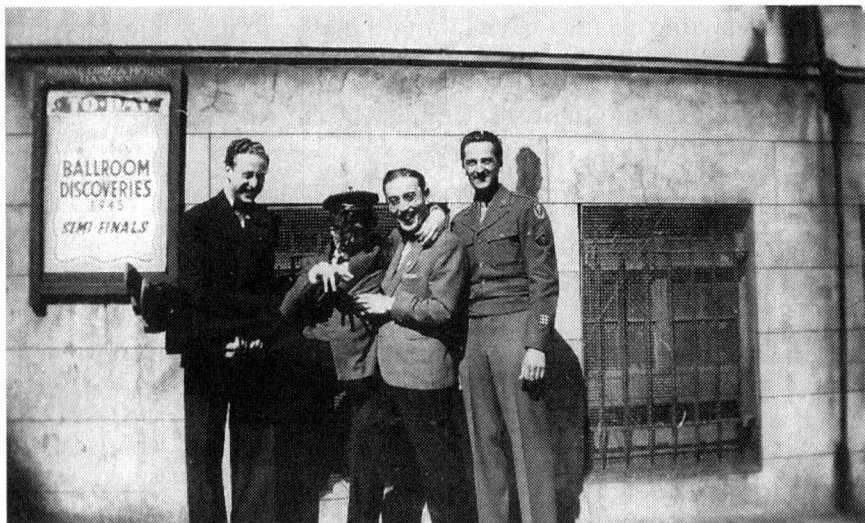

Outside Covent Garden Opera House. Me and pianist Harry Kahn holding up alto man Stanley Lewis. The GI was a great fan of ours

On another occasion my parents had gone away to Brighton for the evening and my brother was home on leave so we decided to have a party. I was playing Covent Garden and every girl I spoke to I invited back home. When I got to the stage door after the show I couldn't believe my eyes as there was about 30 girls waiting for me there. They were a real mixture too as not only were there civilian girls but Canadian Army and ATS ones. I had to order a fleet of minicabs to get them all to Forest Gate but at least I thought my brother would be pleased. When we got home I rang the bell instead of using my key as I wanted to see Bernard's face when he opened the door. He was certainly surprised as 30 girls marched past him in single file:

"What the fuck have you done? We've already got 12 girls here and there's only six of us!"

My 17 year-old eyes had never seen anything like it. There were girls everywhere, in every room, sitting on the stairs drinking and laughing, and all the time the music providing a soundtrack. I have to admit I spent most of the time in my bedroom "entertaining" a seemingly never-ending conveyor belt of young ladies! It was quite a night.

Very early one dark morning a little earlier in the war, I'd accompanied a girl back on the night bus. I lived a couple of stops further on from her so I decided to walk her to her door from the bus and carry on home. We had to walk partly across Wanstead Flats, a very large common area in East London and we ended up doing what comes naturally. The black-out helped to conceal us but as it was early morning, we didn't expect many people to be about anyway. Just as we were getting to the interesting bit there was an excruciating pain across my legs and an angry request from the postman who'd just cycled over me on his way to way to work. He rather impolitely asked that next time I was in a similar situation, could I at least light a fag to show him where we were?

I freely admit that I've had my fair share of fun with the opposite sex and I sowed quite a few wild oats during those wartime years, even though I was a very young man. One thing there certainly wasn't a shortage of during the war was single women and I took full advantage of the fact that a generation of older competitors was away fighting. I've read articles about the level of promiscuity during WWII being high but nothing's come close to describing the reality. The only slight problem we had was getting the alcohol to fuel the parties we held. We usually solved this by inviting a couple of American GIs. They wouldn't need much persuading to come along when there were girls around anyway but more importantly, they seemed to be able to get hold of booze with ridiculous ease.

Somehow I never felt my parents were fully behind my choice of career. They believed being a musician wasn't a serious job as they felt musicians were people who slept late, drank a lot and chased women: they were right with the last three.

Chapter 8
In the Army Now

The fun had to end sooner or later and not long after the end of hostilities I turned 18. That meant I was due for the call-up and, just as expected, within a few weeks I was summoned for my medical. I'd had a heart murmur as a child so I knew I wasn't going to be passed A1 and sure enough, I wasn't. The medic told me there were a couple of options open to me: I was no good for fighting but I could either apply for a desk job or, as the war was now over and front line combatants weren't the main priority, I could enlist in an entertainment unit. Back in Archer Street I heard that a Canadian Army show had come into town and that the band was a bass player down. So I ended up joining the Canadian Army as a 2nd Lieutenant and we were sent to occupied Germany to entertain the soldiers.

I remember the leader of the show was a Canadian called Billy Guest, but time's played her tricks again and I don't recall any of the other names in the troupe apart from the comedian who was a chap called Franklin. We were sent to the British sector and were first stationed in a small town called Bad Zwischenahn but later moved to the town of Delmenhorst near to Bremen. We stayed for about six months in total and each night we were taken out to a different army camp in the area to do the show. Many years later while on business in that part of Germany, I asked my taxi driver if he would mind making a detour into Delmenhorst but he said I would miss my flight because we'd end up stuck in traffic. I was surprised and I told him that when I'd stayed there 35 years earlier it was only a small town but he replied that it certainly wasn't the case now.

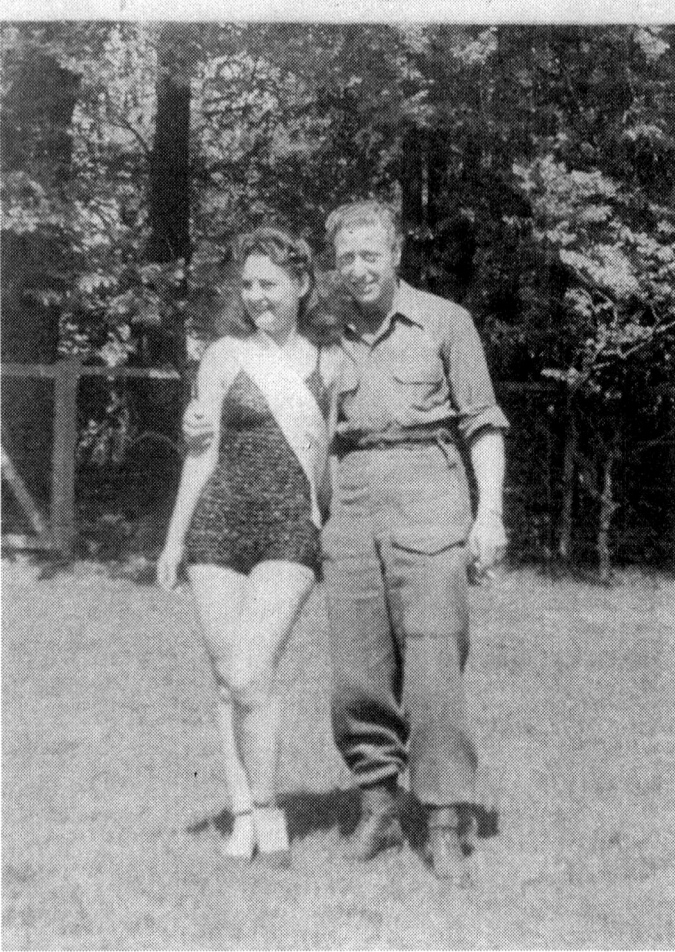

2nd Lieutenant Kaye with a Canadian Beauty Queen in Germany

Rather than the show, the lasting memories of that year concerned different aspects of the devastation the allies had wrought on the country. Many of the large industrial towns had been almost completely razed. One day we went to Bremerhaven and there was hardly a single building standing as far as I could see. The River Weser had almost stopped flowing because it had been dammed by debris from the ruined buildings falling into it.

Not all the damage was physical as the population was also suffering. It had endured a painful and humiliating defeat and now their country was an occupied zone being carved up into administrative areas to be governed by the victors. There was little infrastructure and hardly any industry to provide jobs. The country had been pounded by repeated knockout punches and the Marshall Plan was still a year away. There was an air of desperation about the people that was terrifying at times although being Jewish I wasn't entirely sympathetic, for completely understandable reasons.

One day I was walking around Bad Zwischenahn, smoking a cigarette and looking at the ruined buildings. I was thinking that this is what they'd got for bombing us when I became aware of being followed. I turned round and saw about ten people paying me closer attention than I would otherwise have wished. Thinking I was going to be attacked, I threw my cigarette down and started making a hasty getaway. When I looked back to see if they were still behind me I saw that they were all fighting amongst themselves and I realised that they were actually fighting over my discarded cigarette.

Cigarettes were part of the unofficial black-market currency of Germany. Following their defeat, Germany's own currency, the Reichsmark, was next to useless and the Deutschmark had yet to be introduced. Cigarettes, chocolate, soap and other items, usually obtained from the rations of the occupiers by illegally trading valuable items, had become part of a bartering system.

Bad Zwischenahn is now a flourishing spa town and tourist destination on the banks of a large mere; back then it was a depressing place. The band's drummer and I went into a kind of biergarten and while we were having a drink the owner asked us if we were interested in buying some Solingen steel razors. He brought out a beautiful selection of cut-throats and told us how many cigarettes he wanted for them. While we were looking at them we noticed some suspicious looking characters enter the place. We both decided that we didn't like the look of them and that we had better make a quick exit. We threw down a packet of cigarettes on the table, grabbed two razors and left at the double, showing the blades as we went.

Two days later the bodies of two soldiers were found floating in the lake and we were told that the MPs had raided the biergarten and arrested some suspects who they later found out were ex-gestapo. Later they were proven to have been the murderers. The place was closed down but I still consider we were lucky to get out alive and it was a relief when we were finally transferred to Delmenhorst.

There was a particularly chilling episode one day in Hamburg. Four of us had travelled into the city to indulge in some of the illegal trading with cigarettes we'd heard was carried on there and after we'd finished we went to a beer hall for an ersatz beer. After a while the other guys told me that there was a girl staring intently at me. I looked across and saw they were right; there was indeed a girl there and her eyes were fixed intently on me. I smiled at her and she made her way over to our table. She explained in the little English she had that I was the double of her fiancé. He had been a U-boat commander and she brought out a photo of him, standing in the conning tower of his command. It could have been a picture of myself I was looking at, the likeness was amazing. She then burst into tears saying he'd been killed. I didn't know what to do as there were so many mixed emotions going on. I said to her that I was sorry but at the same time I couldn't help thinking that I was looking at the face of the enemy and wondering how many men he'd killed. Sobbing her heart out, she ran out of the beer hall.

I had "bought" a Leica camera in Hamburg with my cigarettes. Just after I got it, I was approached by a Military Police sergeant and asked whether I knew what I'd done was illegal. Bang to rights! I told him I did and asked him what he was going to do about it. He took me aside and told me I looked a smartarse and asked me my name. When I told him it was Kaye, he asked me whether I'd changed my name. I said no, but that my father had before we were born. He said I was a Luntzman, a fellow Jew.

"Shalom! Let's see how smart you are. We'll wage our own war on these bastards after what they did to us."

He told me to go out and buy everything good I could and to leave the rest to him. I said I didn't have enough cigarettes but he told me not to worry, and again, to leave it to him. I went out and bought another camera, a superb Rolleiflex that used up all my cigarettes. A while later the MP reappeared with my cigarettes. He had been watching the sale and as soon as the seller had gone round the corner he was arrested, cautioned and the cigarettes confiscated. These he gave straight back to me so I could go back out and do it again. This routine went on all day and we ended up with so much stuff we had to find somewhere safe to store it all.

The MP also told me about a guy in Hamburg who was an agent for the rich who were too concerned with their image to want to go out on the street and barter. He'd accumulated a huge horde of valuables and his office was supposedly like an Aladdin's cave. The MP's plan was to break into the place and confiscate all the gear for himself, and for me if I wanted to join him in his endeavour. I agreed. I was 18, game for anything and after all, he was a German so it was retribution again. Moreover, he was a German crook: what could he do? It was all black market gear so he shouldn't have had it anyway and he was hardly going to complain. The MP told me to come back on a certain day and when I did, he was livid. He'd found out four other Canadians had beaten us to it and got away with the lot!

I hadn't got a clue how to use any of the cameras I'd obtained so when we got back to the base I found a local German professional photographer and he taught me all he knew about photography for a couple of packets of cigarettes. He taught me how to use the Leica properly and also how to take, develop and print my own pictures. This was fate playing her hand again; after all, I didn't really know what I was going to do when I got back to England but now I had another skill under my belt. I had an idea!

Chapter 9
Smile Please!

I returned to England early in the Spring of 1946. Always looking out for a way to turn a penny into a pound I decided that photography wasn't going to stay a hobby, it was to be my career. Or at least my next career!

I started by taking pin-up and portfolio pictures for dancers and other showbiz folk I knew. The trouble was, I just couldn't get it right. Usually it was the lighting that was wrong, either too harsh or too soft. Maybe portraiture wasn't my forté so I looked for something that I'd feel more comfortable with. I liked sport so I thought that maybe I could make a decent fist of sports photography. Obviously it was all in natural light and I wouldn't have to bother about poses either so I could take the shots when I felt it was right to. It was much easier!

I went over to West Ham speedway Stadium at Custom House and offered to take some pictures of the riders. I took some individual pictures and also some action shots. I then telephoned the Sporting Pictorial, one of the big sports papers of the day and offered my services as a freelance photographer. They reckoned I was good enough from what they'd seen and said yes.

They'd only been going a few months and it wasn't a brilliant paper but they used to cover greyhound racing, boxing, wrestling and speedway amongst others and there was always a market for picture magazines as this was still way before widespread television sports coverage.

Although I was taking their pictures, I wasn't all that knowledgeable about the sportsmen themselves when I first started out and at the end of a race I used to have to go and ask the winner his name and jot it down! Also, when I went out on a job I wore a big hat just like a movie press-man. I used to carry around a press cutting from a rival magazine that said, "Who was that brash young photographer with the big hat who had the audacity to photograph the riders and then ask their names?" I made a few bob from advertising my pictures for sale in the paper but I was very much an amateur cottage industry as I was still only working out of my bedroom at my parents' house. I was up all night printing usually because I couldn't afford expensive equipment and there was certainly no way I could afford a studio. Something had to happen again soon and like everything else in this story, one thing led on to the next.

All-in or freestyle wrestling was a hugely popular sport post war and I used to go and cover the bouts at West Ham Baths for the Sporting Pictorial. I got to know the promoter very well, a guy called George Callaghan, who also owned a south London baker's shop. One night I took a picture of George Callaghan, his partner George Dingley and the fighter Bert Assirati, apparently discussing Assirati's forthcoming challenge to world title-holder Steve Casey. I sent it to the Sporting Pictorial and they used it on their cover and ran an article inside.

When George Callaghan read the article he asked me if I'd be interested in helping to promote wrestling with him and his partner Dingley, who was a well-known boxing establishment figure at the time from Scotland. When I asked why me especially, he said he thought I would be an asset for their promotional activities. From George Callaghan I learnt all the tricks and wrinkles of the game and eventually started to put on my own promotions. George Dingley wasn't initially all that keen on me being taken on board by the other George but we eventually became friends.

SOCCER ● BOXING ● SPEEDWAY ● GREYHOUNDS ● WRESTLING ● R

★ SPORTING ★

Pictorial

OL. I No. 5   FRIDAY, 27th SEPTEMBER   (PUBLISHED EVERY 4th WEEK)   Price—SIXPENCE

Discussing Wrestling Title Match

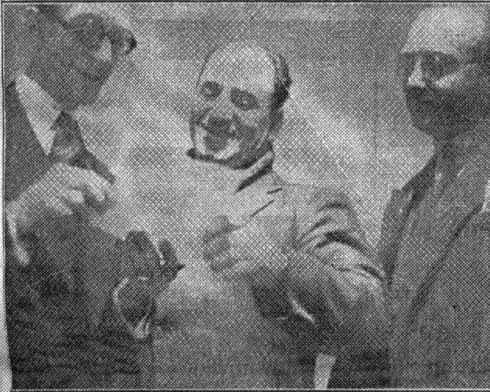

ARSENAL at HO

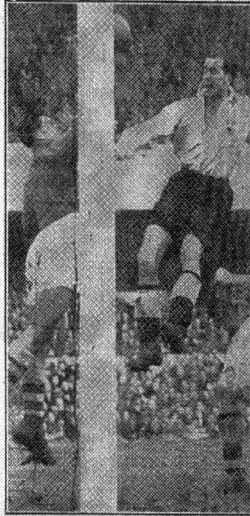

At the famous Highbury ground the Arsenal were at home on Saturday afternoon last. This shot shows Swindin (left), keeper, making a brilliant save from the Derby attacker here the Arsenal defender, is seen on the right.

The Doctor says "NO"

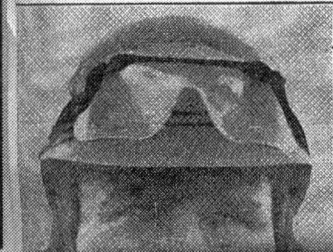

ASSARITI CHALLENGES CASEY

Our cameraman, Tony Kaye, caught Promoter George Callaghan (left) chatting over the details of the proposed world's heavy-weight wrestling championship with challenger Assariti (centre) who hopes to meet champion Steve Casey shortly. George Dingley, the Glasgow promoter, appears most interested in the conversation. Perhaps he has ideas for a return match!

CANADA v ENGl at WEMBLEY Al

First Big Ice Hockey Clash of t

By MARTIN P. THORNTON

THE two new Canadian players, Les Anstice and George Steele, make their debut at Wembley tomorrow evening, when they take the ice for the Canadians against England.

Teams at Full Strength.

The game should prove to be a very interesting one with both teams at full strength, and there will be three pre-war Wembley Juniors, Johnny Murray, Johnny Oxley and Arthur Green playing

against the Las, St lineup.
The teams are as fo England: Jack An Davey, Johnny Mu Arthur Green, A "Red" Townsend, Frankie Green, Ray C Canada: former Duke Campbell, S Scattelood, Freddie Lee, Ivor Smith, Welsh, George Ste

BOB GUINESS LIMIT

Members of the Victoria Club, Na League, National Turf Protecti

The picture I took for the Sporting Pictorial of George Callaghan, Bert Assirati and George Dingley that led to my involvement in wrestling

In the summer of 1946 I met another character who would also have a major, if indirect, influence on my future. The great American lightweight boxer, Ike Williams, a noted puncher and exponent of the "bolo" punch (an extravagantly wide and sweeping uppercut - often a diversionary tactic rather than a punch) was down to fight Welshman Ronnie James for the lightweight championship of the world on

September 4th in Cardiff. I was sent by the Sporting Pictorial to Jack Solomons' gym to photograph Williams training. It was there that I met a guy called "Professor" Jack Robinson, who happened to be a martial arts champion originally from Newcastle but had just come along to see Williams train and spar. We got chatting about this and that and he asked me what paper I worked for. I told him I was a freelance and that I was here taking pictures for the Sporting Pictorial. I also told him that I was getting involved in wrestling promotion. We quickly became friends. In the meantime though, the grapple game took over.

Chapter 10
Grunt and Grapple

I am hugely indebted here to Mike Hallinan of Edgware, London, an expert on wrestling from this era and the biographer of the great Bert Assirati. Meeting Mike while writing this book helped lift the fog clouding my own memories from 50 years ago; it was like having my memory served up to me on a platter and through him I've been able to recall names and link them to events far better than I had been able to before.

-ooOoo-

As I mentioned earlier, wrestling was hugely popular and for me, it proved to be quite a lucrative venture. It also allowed the showman in me to come to the fore, something that's always been a part of my make-up in almost anything I've done. This was one of professional wrestling's golden eras and many of the characters were household names. Remarkable considering that this was still well before the days of televised wrestling. It offered a cheap night's entertainment for everybody; important as things were still very tight for all of us after the war.

Nevertheless, despite the athleticism, the shows were more often than not fixed. Heavyweights were only paid around £10 and lightweights only £4.10.0 (£4.50) a fight and nobody was going to risk serious injury for that kind of money, so entertainment was the order of the day. Sometimes a fighter would be invited to "shoot", that is to fight straight but they were risking serious injury if they did. That injury would be financial as well as physical as no wrestler would want to be out of action too long if he got hurt. While many of the moves looked spectacular, they were all incredibly well-rehearsed and nine times out of ten, each fighter knew what was coming next. They may have looked like lumbering giants but they were skilled performers as well as athletes. Bert Assirati had been a tumbler in a variety act before turning pro so knew how to fall and roll and to make it look convincing. He certainly wasn't the only one.

I promoted all over the south-east from Brighton to London and I can remember planning bills working from George Callaghan's bakery. It could be hectic stuff, too. For instance, we'd put on a show every week at the Rochester roller-skating sink. Such was the fixed nature of the fights, I would put on Tony Mancelli as the bad guy there and then rush him up to West Ham baths the same night where he'd be the good guy!

Even though the fights were fixed, the fighters made it look good and their play-acting could really fire up the crowds. I staged a summer night bill at Brisbane Road, Leyton Orient FC's ground. Top of the card was Jack Pye, from Wigan. He was a man the crowd loved to hate and he was not known as "Dirty" Jack Pye for nothing; on this occasion he certainly lived up to his name, even before he'd got his feet on the canvas. As he walked down to the ring a woman got up and whacked him behind the legs with an umbrella. He turned round, grabbed the brolly and broke it over his knee. The audience went wild and it sounded like they wanted to kill him! They were booing him and giving him the finger but it was all part of the show. He was a genius at working the crowd up but he was a genuinely nice guy outside the ring.

There's nothing more emotive than seeing a bit of blood and I used to use one particular fighter, Chick Knight, whose nose used to bleed very easily, in order to fire the crowd up. When we used him we would always ask for blood in the second round and all his opponent needed to do was rub the palm of his hand on Chick's nose and the blood would flow. The crowd loved it, they thought he was really hurt.

One of my most successful promotions, and the most memorable, was one I put on at Hove Town Hall. A fighter called Abdul the Turk had been acclaimed world champion and had received loads of publicity in the papers and on the newsreels after he came over here in 1947. Questions were even asked in parliament about him after crowds had tried to force their way into a match between him and Bert Assirati at Clapham Baths. He acted the part well; he wore a fez, didn't speak English and was incredibly strong. In short, a guaranteed crowd pleaser.

I managed to book Abdul to fight Tony Mancelli at Hove and we went to work promoting the show. Tickets were sent out to the various agencies and I had fez-wearing sandwich board men walking around Brighton and Hove a week before the match with boards saying that Abdul the Turk was in town. My favourite uncle, Harry, had come down with us and on the day of the fight I got him to take Abdul around town on a tour of the tea shops, the fighter wearing his fez so he'd get noticed. Harry told me that they went to one of the large tea shops and ordered a high tea, which Abdul proceeded to gulp down like he'd never seen food before. Harry also said that as he didn't speak English, he'd been calling him names, all the time with a smile on his face; pleasantries such as "You ugly bastard" and "You pig face". Abdul never said a word, why would he? He *was* Turkish, after all.

Tickets sold like hot cakes and when I arrived on match day the agencies told me they had sold out and were begging me for more. I began to realise just how popular Abdul was and I was starting to think of a possible rematch. When we arrived at the town hall they were queuing round it twice! I went to see the clerk to see if he could let any more punters in but he said it was against fire regulations. I shook his hand, thanking him for his help and palmed him the two £10 notes I'd rolled up and hidden in my hand "just in case". When he held on to the money I knew we were in business. He just told me to be careful how many extras I let in; I was - I managed to squeeze in another 500! That must have been the market training from my father working again.

In case the other heavyweights didn't turn up I'd brought down another wrestler, Battling Phil Siki, who was on leave from the RAF at the time, and sat him in the crowd. When the MC announced the main event, Mancelli vs The Turk, both men came into the ring. Abdul unrolled his prayer mat and got out his compass in order to face East. He got down on his knees and started to pray loudly, at which point the crowd started booing (we weren't very politically correct back then). There was already a great atmosphere brewing but it was to get even better. The MC introduced the grapplers and then announced that Battling Phil Siki had come to watch the Turk fight and was in the crowd. Siki then climbed into the ring to shake hands with the two combatants. He shook Mancelli's hand and went over to Abdul, who had his back to him. Siki tapped Abdul on the shoulder to get him to turn round and shake hands. He did turn round but instead of shaking hands, he suddenly gave Siki a forearm smash. Siki staggered back apparently injured, bringing the crowd to its feet as they sensed blood! The seconds rushed in to keep Siki back and as they escorted him from the ring he was shouting "I'll get you! So help me, I will!"

The match went on and Abdul the Turk won after a very dirty fight. We then had the MC climb into the ring to announce that we had spoken to Phil Siki's commanding officer and he had been granted a 24 hour pass to come and fight the Turk in two weeks time. Tickets would be available on the way out! What was that about it all being stage managed? I was giving the punters what they wanted and it was the modest start of the elaborate play acting and stage management that we see on TV today.

At the end of the evening the wrestlers were coming in to be paid. Uncle Harry was with me and when Abdul the Turk came in I tried to give him £12.

"I've wrestled for £15, you know that." He said in a broad Canadian accent. "He speaks English!" Whimpered Uncle Harry as the blood drained from his face.

"Yeah, and if you want to call me a pig faced bastard again, I'll put you in a head-lock!" Abdul was about as Turkish as I was!

The four of us, Abdul, Tony Mancelli, Uncle Harry and myself had driven to Brighton in my brother's broken down old Vauxhall and on the way back we needed some petrol and desperately needed some oil. We stopped at a garage but it was closed. We banged on the door until eventually a man appeared at a window and put a light on. He looked down to see these huge blokes with cauliflower ears looking up at him.

"We want oil," said Abdul. "If you won't give us any, we'll take it." At which point he went over to the garage door and broke the padlock open. The owner just looked at him and choked, "You want more?" We filled up with petrol and oil but we only got as far as Elephant and Castle, where we got a puncture. My efficient brother had guaranteed that we wouldn't have a jack with us so the two wrestlers were pressed into service to lift up the back of the car while we changed the wheel. It must have been quite a sight.

Other wrestlers I had working for me included the Lipman Brothers, who were two lightweight Jewish brothers from Aldgate; Giant Anaconda and Big Bill Benny. Poor Bill had trouble saying the letter "S" and he also had a long beard. One night we got Tony Mancelli to tie Bill's beard in the ropes and give him repeated forearm smashes. Unfortunately the beard got knotted up and poor old Bill was shouting, "Tony! Shilly boy, shtop!" In the end we had to cut him out with scissors and needless to say, the crowd loved it! Bill ended up a successful businessman owning nightclubs and sporting clubs around Manchester. One of his club MCs was Bernard Manning. I also had Jan Dale with me. He used to fight for £4.10.0 (£4.50) a time but then went on to form the hugely successful Dale Martin Promotions.

After a while disillusionment began to set in and I was starting to get a bit tired of the shenanigans that were going on. Some of the guys had formed a federation and wanted me to become their chairman but their own activities were in danger of cutting their own throats commercially. For instance, Issy van Dutz, a huge and popular 22 stone Dutchman, who also had ideas about being my minder, was often to be seen in the bar before fights knocking back whiskies. If this was going on, how on earth could the public even begin to believe that what we were serving up was anything but contrived?

My announcer, Sammy King, wanted me to go in with him and form a promotions company (he was successful too, and would later put on bouts for television). I though had been mulling over another suggestion made some time earlier by Jack Robinson, which was to go and promote wrestling in South Africa, where he now lived. Wrestling was almost unknown there and there was a market ripe for exploitation using our own roster of fighters. And the longer I thought about it, the more attractive a proposition it seemed to be.

Post-war Britain was depressing. Rationing was still in operation and I was becoming fed up with it. It wasn't only food that was being rationed either; you couldn't even get a double-breasted suit because it used too much cloth. A tailor in the East End used to make our double-breasted suits for us and he said that every time he heard a knock on the door his heart would sink into his boots because he thought it was the police. When you went for a fitting he used to bring the suit out of hiding for you to try on and then when you collected it you had to rush out with the package under your arm, hoping you weren't going to get stopped. If you were, you then had to make up a story about you being given the suit by a friend who was now too fat for it! In fact, I have a picture of Jack Robinson and myself in my parents' garden and in it I'm wearing one of those "illegal" suits!

No, it seemed rationing would never end and avoiding it by moving away was a great solution so, in early 1948, I took the momentous decision to up sticks and leave for South Africa. I knew I was going to be a very long way from home and I'd only know Jack out there but I was already a seasoned traveller of 5 years experience so I wasn't too bothered by the extra distance. I also reasoned that my mother would be fine now that my brother was back at home, a fact that made the decision to go that much easier. I booked my passage and I was away!

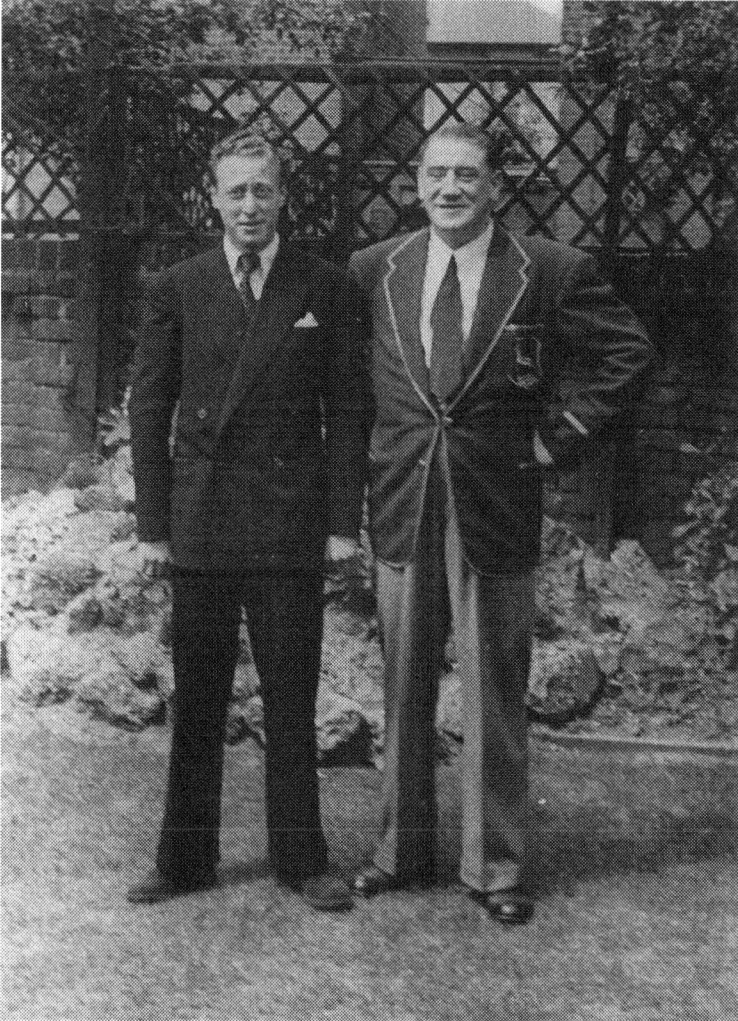

Myself, left, and Jack Robinson. I'm wearing an "illegal" suit

Chapter 11
Heading South

I could have sailed down to South Africa but the trip would have taken two weeks and I didn't want to waste time, so I decided to fly. Intercontinental air-travel wasn't taken for granted like it is today and long haul flights were much more of an adventure. The BOAC DC4's flight down to Johannesburg from London took in 3 stopovers, Tripoli in Libya, Khartoum in The Sudan and Kasama in Zambia and it lasted for 36 stifling and exhausting hours. What's more, in time-honoured fashion, the airline had managed to lose my baggage in London, so all I had with me were the clothes I stood up in. On the same flight were the Great Britain Cycling team and General Wavell, who had until recently been Viceroy of India.

At the halfway stop we were offered the chance of a bath. Even though I didn't have a change of clothes with me, we'd been in the air for over 16 hours and I jumped at the chance. Stood outside the bathroom was a huge black guy wearing what I thought was a nightshirt, a fez and carrying a bloody great sword! I needn't have been afraid, he was in fact a guard very thoughtfully provided by BOAC to prevent me being taken advantage of while I was luxuriating in the water.

At the final stopover before Johannesburg I decided I needed a shave. I always used to use an electric razor but that had been lost with my luggage so I sought out a barber at the airport. I eventually found one and settled back for a shave. I must have been exhausted and half-asleep because all I can remember was the barber lathering me up and beginning to shave me. When I got back to the plane there was a gasp from the stewardess as she asked me what had happened.

I was covered in plasters and I was so tired that I'd not noticed anything. I think I must have had Sweeney Todd's apprentice.

It was winter when we left London but when we arrived in Jo'burg of course it was sweltering mid-summer - and I was still in my winter clothes. And of course then I had to wait another four days for my luggage to catch up with me.

I was met by Jack Robinson and went to stay with him and his family. After discussing Jack's ideas about promoting wrestling there I soon came to the conclusion that it was a non-runner. He was expecting the guys to stump up the cost of their fares to South Africa and in the 40s, air travel was considered a luxury and well beyond the means of the average man in the street. Now I was going to have to tell Jack that wrestlers being paid £10 a fight were not going to be able to finance their own passage and that his grandiose ideas were next to unworkable. I would have to back out. I knew this would not be what Jack would want to hear and I was also concerned that here I was, 6000 miles from home, on a bit of a wild goose chase, with nowhere to go once my reason for being there had now been removed.

Jack's son, Joe, was a magnificent specimen of manhood and I had a flash of inspiration that I thought might just help to temper the blow of my pulling out. Joe was blond and built like the proverbial outhouse but with a waist a woman would kill for. Like his Dad, he was also a martial arts expert. His Greek god looks and physique told me he could have a chance in the movies so I suggested to them that Joe should go to London and meet up with some of the agents there. To my surprise they immediately forgot about the wrestling and started questioning me about whether I really did think he had a chance.

I must have been convincing because he did indeed go and I was proven right, too. He studied at RADA and starred in several high profile movies including "A Kid for Two Farthings" alongside Diana Dors and "Diamonds Are Forever" in which he fought with Sean Connery's James Bond in the famous elevator scene. He's now retired to the south of England but in 1998 and at the age of 70 his still action-man like physique and immense strength came to his aid. On a visit to Cape Town, South Africa, he was attacked by a gang of eight muggers but he managed to successfully fight them off, poleaxing a few with drop-kicks and karate chops and breaking another's arm before the rest ran away. A formidable man indeed.

Not wishing to impose on the Robinsons' hospitality for too long I checked in to a local hotel. After leaving my luggage in my room I decided to go out and explore the city. My eyes nearly popped out of my head as I gazed upon shops crammed with all those things we'd been deprived of in Britain for nearly a decade. I went into a shop that sold fruit and sweets and which also had a juice bar selling milk shakes. I ordered a chocolate milkshake and gulped it down – I was in heaven! I then stocked up on oranges, peaches, bananas and a huge box of chocolates to take back to my room. I'm sorry to say I gorged on all these forgotten luxuries until I was ill. I would also soon discover tropical fruits and treats that I and presumably nobody from England had ever heard of before, like passion fruit, mangoes and guavas. This really was paradise on earth and the true land of plenty.

Living in a hotel, I was soon going to run out of money if I didn't find work very quickly. I was a stranger in a foreign city though, what did I do now? I knew I had a relation in the city somewhere but I didn't know their name. I phoned my parents and found out that it was one of my father's cousins and that her married name was Mantel. I looked in the phone book and there were only 5 Mantels listed so I started to call them. I hit the jackpot on number 3 and when they heard who their mystery caller was they invited me round to dinner the following night.

She'd done very well for herself; her husband owned a large used car showroom and they lived in a beautiful house in a wealthy suburb of Johannesburg. They also had two children of around my own age, a boy and girl. As we all sat down to dinner I had my first real introduction to a different social system: we were waited upon by a black guy all dressed in white.

After dinner, the son and daughter asked me if I wanted to go on to a nightclub. As I had nothing else planned, I agreed and it turned out to be a fortuitous night out for me. The place was called The Orange Grove and the bandleader was a chap called Roy Martin. In the interval I went over to him and introduced myself, telling him that I was a bass player. He told me that it just so happened they needed a bass player for their recordings and broadcasts as his vocalists only held the bass for show during performances and couldn't play it. I said I didn't have a bass with me but he said that was no problem as I could use his. So much for the wrestling, I was back playing music again.

I think I must have impressed Roy because I remember he set me up as an example to the rest of the band when we were playing a scored orchestration of a Glenn Miller piece that had an intricate four-bar bass intro. I played it fine but the band never came in when they were meant to because they were all looking at me aghast! Roy, in his terribly pukka accent berated them: "Look at you, you're all wondering "How?" He sight-read because he has training, gentlemen and that's what you all need!" I would stay working with Roy most of the time I was in South Africa.

In that first session I did with Roy Martin I met other session musicians who helped me to get other nightclub work and within a few months I was working full time as a musician. I was also earning enough to cash to get my own instrument on hire purchase. Coincidentally, it was an American-made Kay (so I was a Kaye with a Kay) and also a very unusual 5-string model that took a little bit of time to get used to. I also had enough to get a flat in the centre of town. I couldn't believe my luck as yet again, after a bad start, I appeared to have fallen straight back firmly onto my feet.

I never seemed to be short of work. First were the daytime broadcasts Roy Martin hired me to perform on. These were from the studios of the South African Broadcasting Corporation. I would also work full time with Roy about four years later. I then went on to play full time with tenor sax man Don Barrigo at the Stork Club. I was still able to do the broadcasts so I was doing OK.

The Stork club was quite an eventful place. One night I was playing and there was a group of "Yaapies" sitting at a table directly under my position on the bandstand. One guy kept taunting me, calling me a "Bloody rooineck" this being the derogatory name the Boers used for the British army soldiers after the sunburn they used to get, rooineck meaning "red neck" in Afrikaans. This taunting went on for an hour or so and I had just about had enough of it by the time we finished playing. He had his hand stretched out on the table in front of him and I picked up my bass and jabbed the metal pointed stabilising peg protruding from the bottom of the instrument directly between his thumb and forefinger:

"I may well be a rooineck" I told him, "But I certainly won't be taking any more of that shit and if you don't shut up, next time I might not be so accurate."

He said he was sorry and that he was only teasing me and could he buy me a drink? I thought why not, he was buying after all so I joined them. I got chatting to a pretty young girl at their table and ended up making a date with her. A few months later and she was making headlines in the national papers as the victim in a strange murder case. Her name was Jacoba "Bubbles" Schroeder and the case has remained a veritable mystery since that day in August 1949 when she was found in the Birdhaven Plantation, apparently asphyxiated by a ligature. A piece of hard clay-like earth had been placed in her mouth after her death, which was a common thing to do among some African peoples in order to prevent the victims of violent crime talking about it in the afterlife. However, it seemed she had been killed and deliberately placed where she was discovered and the object placed in her mouth as a possible decoy.

Nobody was convicted of her murder although I had my own theory regarding the manner of her death in that it was a sexual act that went badly wrong, although the post mortem evidence appeared not to back this up. I also had my own ideas as to who the killer was and that he evaded prosecution because of corrupt evidence. Either way, it was a terrible tragedy. To this day the Bubbles Schroeder case is thought of as South Africa's most famous unsolved murder.

While doing the broadcasts with Roy, I met Dick Norton. He was preparing a jazz show to go on air and asked me if I'd like to take part in that, too. Dick would later go on to become a well known radio voice in the UK where he was an announcer on Radio Luxembourg and also the German "link" on World Wide Family Favourites. It was while doing these broadcasts that I also met Dave Lee and Herbert Kretzmer. We became great friends and played together often, with Dave and I having regular Sunday night jazz sessions at the Jewish Guild. Herbie wrote the following in a review published in one of the local newspapers:

"I like Tony Kaye's bass work. When given the sign, he can make his digits buzz and blur like any virtuoso, but, for the main part, he appreciated that the bass was a workmanlike and rather unglamorous instrument..."

He goes on to mention Andy Johnson, the drummer, with whom I used to duet on "Big Noise From Winnetka": "[the duet]...gave them both the chance to show off their technical expertise, a chance they grabbed (literally) with both hands."

This last part refers to the fact that Andy used to play a solo on the G string of my bass with his sticks in the manner made famous by Ray Baudoc and Bob Haggart, who wrote the song.

I've another old cutting from the same era which says: "Tony always gives of his best and was a sensation at a five piece jam session which I put on at the theatres in Johannesburg." I don't know who wrote it but I must have impressed him!

Both Herbie and Dave would continue to have great careers in music, often working together such as on the comedy songs they did for Peter Sellers ("Goodness Gracious Me" and "Bangers and Mash") and the stage show "Our Man Crichton". Herbie also penned the English libretto for "Les Miserables" while Dave co-founded the London based all-jazz radio station, Jazz Fm. For my part, I was voted No.1 double bass player in South Africa. Although this was a great honour, in fairness there wasn't a lot of competition! Looks like we all eventually did pretty well for ourselves in our chosen fields!

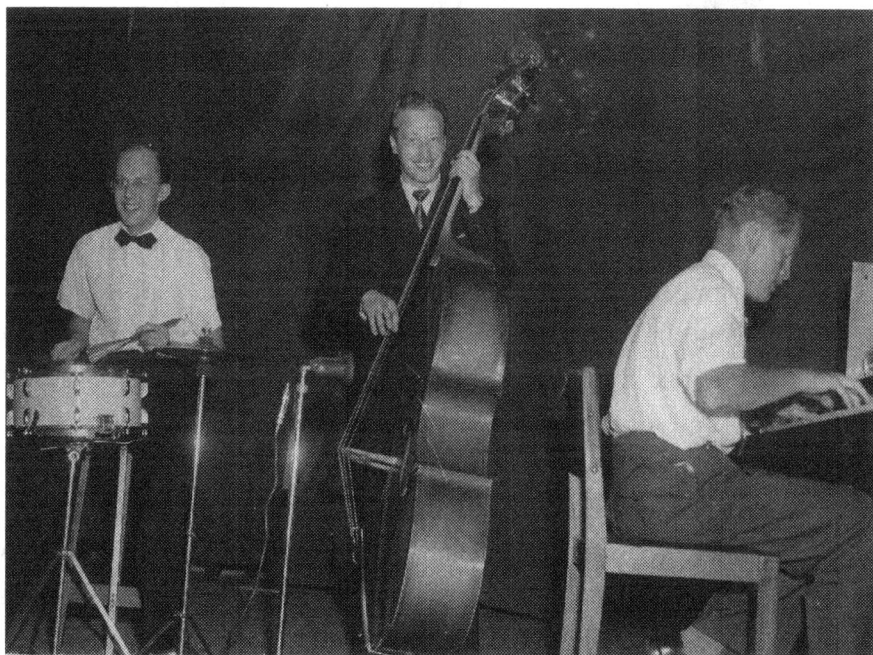

South Africa's No 1 Bass Player!

Following the jazz show, Dave Lee, myself and drummer Andy Johnson were contracted to do a series of recordings for Australian radio. Following on from that, myself, trumpeter Jimmy Lonie, pianist Jack Dent (both from the Stork Club) plus a few others formed another band and this one we took down to Margate on the southern Natal coast where we'd secured a contract at the Margate Hotel.

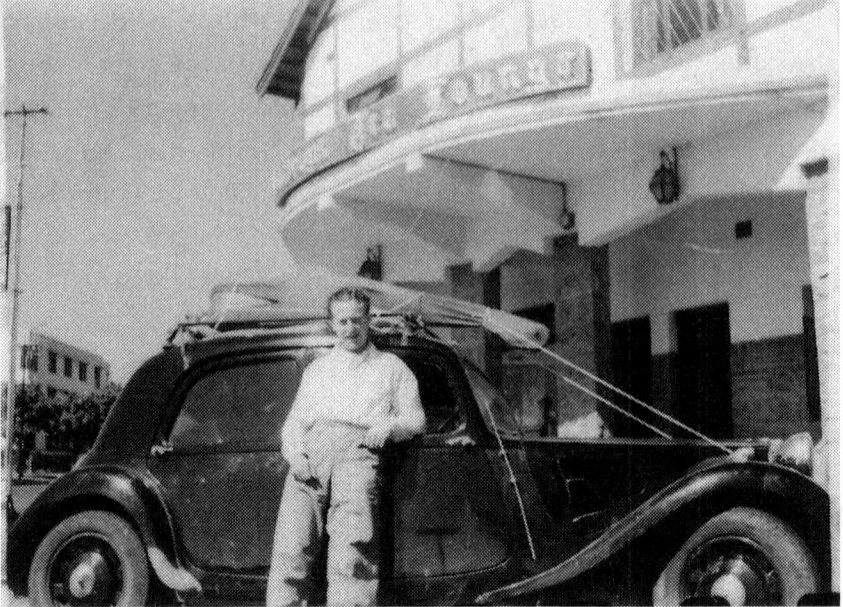

Off to Margate with the bass strapped to the roof of my Citroen

The Margate Hotel was owned by the O'Connor family, also originally from the East End of London. They'd previously owned the well-known Black and White Milk Bar chain and some cinemas back in London. They sold these to Granada and moved out to South Africa on the proceeds. Margate was a sleepy "dorp" when they arrived and they thought it was a bit crazy that the Margate Hotel was at one end of the town and the bank at the other with nothing in-between. They built a small arcade halfway along and all the shops moved there. Now it's a thriving city and tourist resort and one of the main streets is even named after William O'Connor.

They were certainly a no-nonsense family, the grandmother especially. One night while I was there she'd called time in the bar. This had upset the two "yaapies" still in there, who called her a "bloody cow" for her trouble.

"Never mind cow, if I 'ad a pair of bleedin' 'orns I'd ram 'em up yer arse. Now piss orf!" They didn't hang about.

We were asked to put on a show every Sunday night but none of us had ever had any experiencing of writing and producing a show before. I'd at least played in stage shows so the other two gave me the job of putting one together. I worked up a two-hour show that would include a talent show, competitions and a few sketches to keep the holidaymakers happy. I would need to be a bit of a jack of all trades because as well as writing the show I'd have to rehearse it, compère it and also act and play in it. This would all prove to be invaluable experience for later on in my career.

One Sunday afternoon I was sitting on the beach trying to think up new ideas for the next week's show when a huge dog came up to me. I was eating a bar of chocolate at the time and the dog was determined to get it off me. I was in no mood to argue with such a massive beast so I gave him the chocolate and carefully patted his head. He must have liked me as he decided to sit down beside me. I was able to take a closer look now and he appeared to be a cross between a Rhodesian Ridgeback and a Great Dane. It was soon time to go to the theatre for the evening show so I patted him on the head one last time and left.

During the show the audience suddenly started laughing for no reason whatsoever. Nothing funny was scripted and nobody had cocked up, so why? I looked down at my feet and there was this huge dog looking up at me, wagging his tail. I didn't quite know what to do; I could hardly push him off the stage, he was far too big. Thinking fast, I introduced him to the audience as my bodyguard. No name though! Help! Our cat's name back in London was Jackson so the dog very quickly went by the same name:

"Meet Jackson, he's here to protect my honour, something it's very difficult to do here in Margate!"

He stayed on stage for the rest of the show. After we finished I took a look at his collar and found a name and telephone number on it. I rang the number and the owner said that he was in fact a guard dog on their farm but could I look after him overnight and they'd come and fetch him in the morning. The next morning I was walking

Jackson back to the hotel to meet his owners. Coming the other way was a black guy carrying a plank of wood, just going about his business. In a flash, Jackson jumped on him and brought him to the ground with his huge teeth on his neck. The poor man was terrified and so was I. In desperation I shouted for the dog to come to me and to my relief he climbed off his victim and ran back to me. I apologised to the man, giving him a bit of money to smooth over any bad feelings and we went on our way. When I told the owners what had happened they weren't surprised; he was a trained guard dog and would attack anyone who looked to him as though they were going to attack his master. He'd obviously taken to me if he thought I was his master.

The following Sunday we were in the middle of the show doing a sketch in which we played gangsters, sitting round a table discussing a hit. The sketch went pretty well but as the punchline was delivered it was immediately followed by the unlikely sound of something heavy and metal being thrown around as Jackson, dragging half his kennel behind him, came careering into the club. It was a hard act to follow. I phoned the owners again that night who said they'd had to chain him to the kennel as they were wondering what on earth I'd done as I seemed to have had an effect on him. They asked whether I wanted to keep him but I said it was impossible as I would be returning to Jo'burg in a few weeks so they came and once again took him away. He had a sad ending. He had obviously become attached to me as just before I returned to Jo'burg, the owners told me he wouldn't eat anything, he just laid on the floor pining until he wasted away. I never found that depth of love in either of my two marriages.

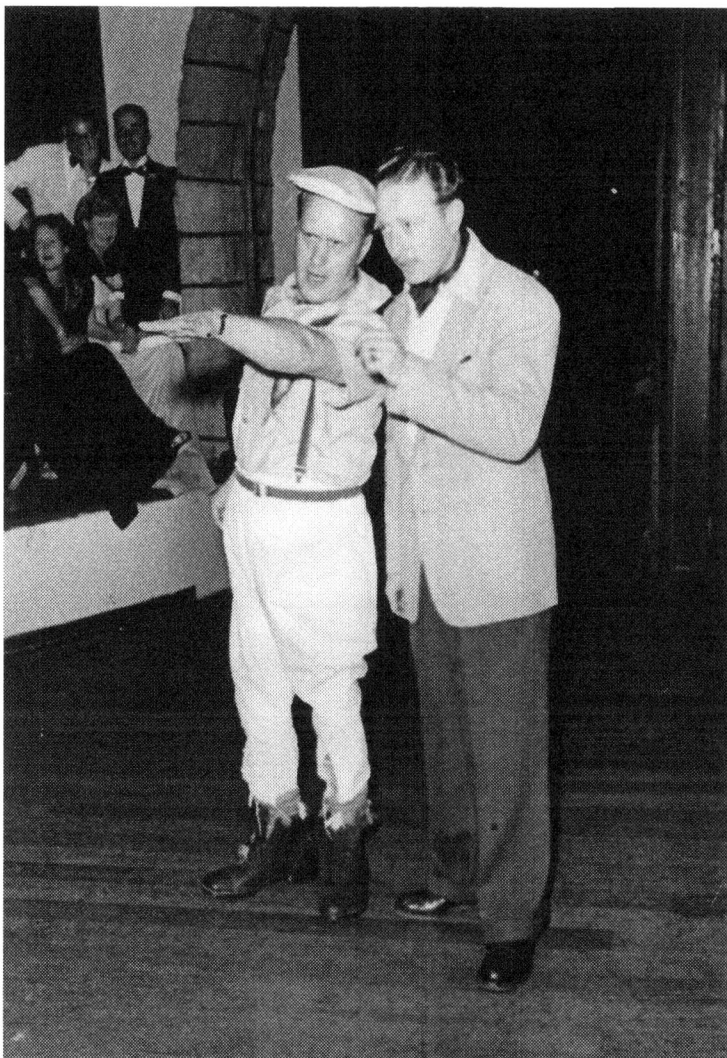

Albert O'Conner and myself in a skit about golf. The O'Connors just about ran
Margate

Chapter 12
Up, Up and Away!

I became aware that in South Africa I was mixing with a very varied group of people from many different backgrounds, not just musicians. When I'd arrived I was a cocky so-and-so who thought he knew it all but I soon realised that if I didn't buck my ideas up I'd soon look out of my depth. I bought a concise English dictionary and every time I heard or read a word I didn't know, I looked it up. In fact, my thirst for knowledge was unquenchable and there wasn't anything I thought was beyond me. Moreover, I was willing to have a go at most things, however unusual they may have seemed.

It was while in Margate that I became interested in hypnosis, devouring book after book on the subject. My mother even went to Foyles in the Charing Cross Road and bought books on it to send out to me. I was itching to try it out on someone so I collared the cleaner of the apartment building I was staying in and told him I was going to try and hypnotise him. I sat him down in an armchair and started talking to him in order to put him under when suddenly he started snoring. It wasn't my doing either, he was fast asleep! Probably because he'd been up since the crack of dawn and this was the first chance of a rest he'd had all day.

I gradually got better at it though. Nobody ever tried it out on me or taught me, I taught myself purely from the books I read. The local doctor was a delightful Jewish chap by the name of Solly Feinberg and I would discuss hypnotism with him while we played chess together whenever I visited him and his wife at their home. We wondered long about the possibility of age regression and how the subconscious mind worked. Desperate to try out some theories, I looked for a willing subject. I found one in a local lifeguard, a real man-mountain of about 20 years old. I lugged him along to Solly's surgery and said I'd like to try out some age regression on him.

I got him under nicely but Solly wanted to do his own test to satisfy himself that he was in a trance state. He asked me to tell the subject that the back of his neck was numb and that he wouldn't be able to feel anything there. So I did, at which point Solly picked up a bloody great needle and stuck it in the bodyguard's neck! He took the needle out and the skin just closed up, no blood or anything. The guy didn't feel a thing and Solly was convinced. I, on the other hand, almost passed out.

We started on the age regression. I told him that I wanted him to show me what position he was in when he was in his mother's womb. At this, the huge guy went into the foetal position. I then asked him what it felt like when he was born and he replied that he was afraid because everything had been all nice and warm and suddenly there were bright lights everywhere. We also asked him what presents he had for his first birthday and he described everything he received. His mother later confirmed to us that he did indeed receive the presents he described. It doesn't seem an exhaustive test by the standards we're used to today but we were convinced there was something in it.

Many people are scared of hypnosis because they are uneasy about somebody controlling them while in a trance. The long and the short of it is that the sub-conscious mind won't let a subject do anything he or she doesn't want to do so the subjects set their own boundaries that the hypnotist couldn't cross if he tried.

Solly said he had a patient who desperately wanted to give up smoking because she felt it was harming her health (this was in the days before the proven links between smoking and cancer, heart disease etc.) and would I be interested in seeing her? I told him that as long as it was fine with her, I would be delighted to try and help her. I went to see her in her home and the first thing that struck me before we started any treatment was that she had a bit of a cast in her left eye.

I asked her about it and she replied that that she was waiting for some corrective surgery. But I'd already had another idea.

I asked her whether I could see if she would make a good subject for hypnosis and if so, would she like me to try an experiment on her eye at the same time as stopping her from smoking. Surprisingly, she agreed to go the whole nine yards.

As far as anatomy was concerned I was a complete ignoramus. All I knew how to do was to hypnotise people, I didn't know anything about the musculature or the structure of the eye. I was confident (and probably too cocky) enough to think I could cure anything so I thought about it and suggested to her under hypnosis that the muscles in her eye were tightening up and that her eye was moving back into its correct position. Whether it was more by luck than judgement, something must have gone right because when she came out of the first session she looked towards a vase on the table in her hall and cried out, "Oh my God! I can see the petals on that flower!"

I was surprised too as I could see that her eye had changed position slightly. We persevered and after just four sessions her eye had returned to its normal position. Even her surgeon was convinced it had worked and he cancelled the corrective surgery he'd planned. I don't know how long the effect lasted but it certainly didn't revert to the cast position while I was there. Of course, once the news about my miracle cure got out, word soon went round Margate that I was a healing man and I had no shortage of customers. Now I was finding it difficult to manage playing music and doing hypnotism at the same time.

I returned to Johannesburg as soon as the work in Margate finished and there I received a letter from my mother telling me she missed me and that she was going to visit. She'd never undertaken such a long journey on her own before and I was worried she might not be able to cope with it but she did. She sailed for two weeks on a Union Castle Line ship from Southampton to Cape Town and then took the famous Blue Train to Jo'burg. I'd got a job playing at a place called the BBQ

Ranch between Johannesburg and Pretoria. It was also where I lived and I booked us both into a two-roomed bungalow there for her stay. She didn't like it though. Being out in the country she couldn't stand the spiders and all the other creepy-crawlies that used to visit during the night. Of course, I was already used to them but I still thought I'd better look for somewhere else for her to stay.

We knew a doctor, originally from London but now living in Jo'burg with his family and luckily they invited mother to stay with them for the rest of her holiday. She settled in and was much happier but after a few days she began to feel ill. The doctor couldn't find anything wrong with her so he called in a specialist but he was also stumped. Her temperature was very high and we were becoming increasingly worried as the fever dragged on. Undeterred, the specialist examined her again and on looking between two toes he saw a tiny puncture wound that he said looked like a tick bite.

He deduced she had tick-bite fever, which is carried by ticks that feed on cattle and that she would have to go on to antibiotics immediately. Back then these were exceedingly expensive, about £1 per pill, as they were still a very new treatment but, they worked well and much to my intense relief, she quickly recovered. Goodness knows what that £1 is equivalent to nowadays but I would have paid anything to help her and if I'd not had the money, I would have got it from somewhere. Maybe she was justified in her fear of the bugs after all. As a treat I decided to drive her and my uncle to Durban in my car, a Chevrolet, so she could see some of the other sights of South Africa.

The BBQ Ranch was owned by a real character called Tommy Ellis, who was an alcoholic. When he was sober he was one of the nicest guys you could meet but like so many drinkers, when he'd had a few, he was unpredictable and you stayed well out of his way, mainly for your own safety.

He kept a pet baboon. He was exceedingly fond of him and on his binges would often get into his cage and drink with him. One day a veterinary inspector visited the ranch to check all the livestock and informed Tommy that the animal was high-risk rabies and if he escaped could be devastating to other animals and humans and would therefore have to be put down. Tommy refused point blank to let anyone but himself put the animal down but he was also absolutely beside himself with grief at having to lose his friend, so he went on a three-day bender. When he returned he climbed into the baboon's cage with a crate of beer and a bottle of brandy and they both drank until they passed out. Next morning, as Tommy wasn't around, we went looking for him. We found the baboon asleep on the empty crate with Tommy's arms embracing him. There was nothing we could do until he came round. Later in the morning the sound of gunshots sent us running to the cage to be met with the sight of Tommy crying over the body of his friend laying at his feet.

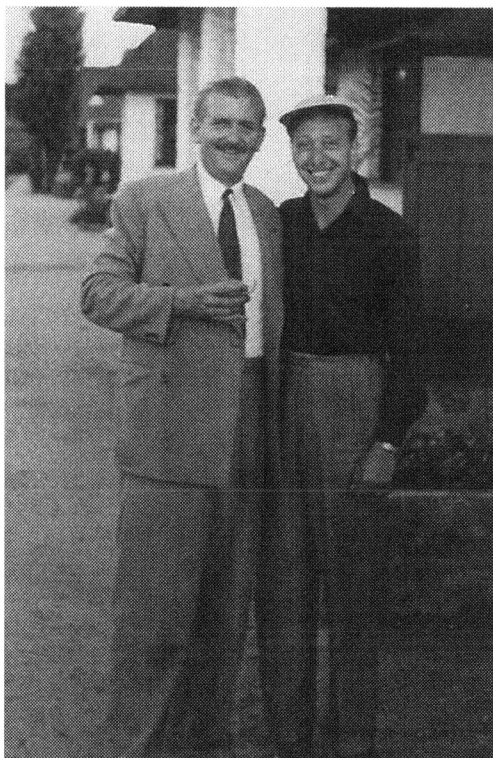

Tommy Ellis, left

Tommy certainly was one of those larger than life characters you hear about now and again that would probably be more at home in a book. He was one of the last white hunters, if you'll forgive the phrase, but that's how he behaved. He was a crack shot but could scare the life out you because of it. I actually introduced him to his future wife and he fell madly in love with her at first. After a while though he'd play a rather terrifying game with her when he was drunk, ordering her to dance while he fired at the ground around her feet with his revolvers. Needless to say, the marriage didn't last.

South Africa was a land of endless possibilities if you were adventurous enough and that description certainly suited me. I really was game for anything and it was while I was at the BBQ that I developed two new passions, namely flying and horse-riding.

Me being me, I didn't just take up flying because I fancied it, there had to be a decent excuse to do something like that and just like almost every other man of my age driven to do anything slightly out of the ordinary, the excuse was invariably female. Yes, I initially took up flying because I was trying to impress another girl I'd fallen in love with back in London. She had worked at Ciro's Night Club and they had decided to start their own airline so they'd bought a Dakota and started flying to Jo'burg with her as the stewardess. It didn't work out but I carried on flying nevertheless and my pilot's licence was granted on St Valentine's Day, 1949 only a year or so after I first arrived in the country. I stopped flying when I got back to England because I couldn't afford it and even after I started making a bit of money I never seemed to have the time for it so I never really gave it another thought. Even so, I loved it for those few years when I was able to fly in the empty wide-open skies of South Africa. It was such a liberating experience.

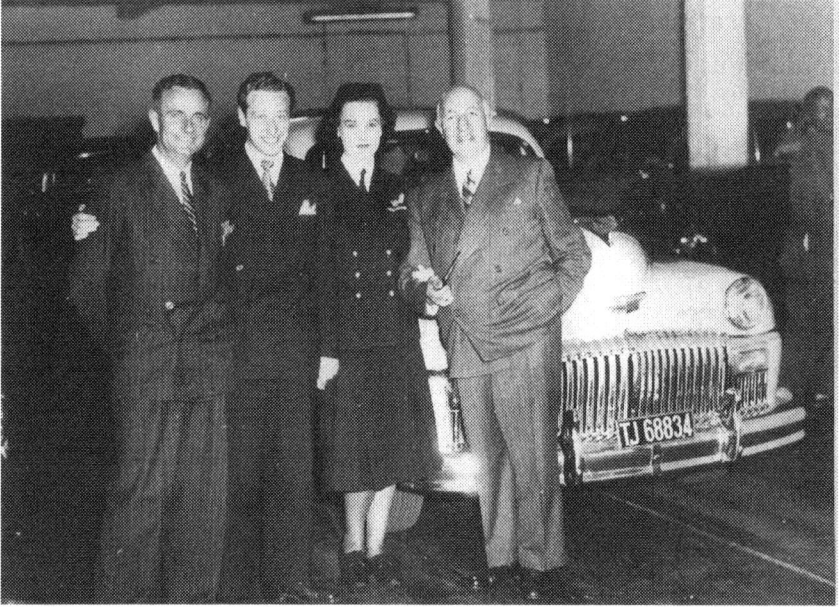

In my Uncle Ben's car showroom with his partner, Syd, on the left, myself and the girl I took up flying to impress. The car behind Ben is a DeSoto and I seriously coveted it

I think I had three different instructors while I was learning, the last one glorying in the name of "Saboteur"! Once during a lesson he remarked that my flying record so far showed I hadn't done any spins. He was right, I hadn't. He suggested that there was no time like the present to learn so he asked me to fly up to 4000 ft so we could do a few. Well, the plane I was flying was a little Aeronca Champion, a tiny but popular plane and often used by flying schools. It was powered by a meagre 60hp engine and Sam, the instructor, was a very heavy man. His weight meant we didn't have enough power to climb to 4000ft so he suggested we look for some thermals, which are the rising columns of warm air on which birds and gliders soar, in order to help us climb.

It's not difficult to find thermals in a hot country and when we got to the required altitude Sam asked, "Do you know what causes a spin?"

"Sam, I have no idea. I thought that's why we're up here."

Now bear in mind we were sitting tandem, with him behind me so I couldn't see what he was going to do with his set of controls. This meant I had absolutely no inkling of what was going to happen next.

"Well, a spin is caused by two things happening. First, you stall the plane and lose airspeed and secondly, you lose control of turning so the plane goes into a spin." Without warning, he pulled the nose of plane right up, put the engine into idle and went into a dive. Then he kicked on left rudder and we started to spin round and round. I was hanging on for dear life yet he was quite calm and telling me what we had to do to recover from a spin like the one we were in.

"First we have to stop the spin, so we have to kick the opposite rudder down hard. So kick the rudder hard to the right to stop the spin. When you've got it rectified you've got to pull the nose back slowly to come out of the dive."

By the time we recovered from that exercise I was completely drenched in sweat and exhausted from a combination of exertion and fear.

"OK, we'll go up again then."

"Do we have to?"

"If you want your licence, you're going to have to learn to control this thing. 4000ft. Now!"

But it's like everything else in life, once you've done it a few times it becomes second nature and I soon got the hang of it.

A couple of important things I couldn't get the hang of for quite a while after I began my lessons were taking-off and landing, I think this was mainly because we were using a grass airstrip all of the time. Also, the Champion was a three-point aircraft with a tail wheel and not a tricycle style with a nose wheel. This means that you start on the ground with your nose facing upwards, looking at the sky and not really looking where you're going. As you gain speed one has to push the stick forward in order to bring the tail up. When it's raised, you're then bouncing across a grass field on two wheels, which is something I found very difficult to control and I usually ended up zig-zagging across the airfield instead of going in a straight line. When you finally got in the air, you'd do your turns and then come in to land.

I'd been doing these "circuits and bumps" for what seemed like ages when Sam, my instructor suddenly ordered, "Taxi to the clubhouse." I thought the lesson had been cut short.

When we got there I started to take my safety belt off but Sam interrupted me. "No, you're not getting out, I am." And with that, he took his belt off and climbed out of the aircraft.

'What do you mean?'

'You're going solo'

'Don't be silly, Sam. I'll kill myself!'

'Don't worry, the plane's insured.'

Well, I could hardly chicken out after paying for all these lessons so I taxied out and for once, took off perfectly. I climbed to 400 ft, turned, climbed to 800 ft and turned again and thought this was great – I was flying solo at last. Then I realised I'd got up there OK but how on earth was I going to get down again? Luckily, everything I'd been taught came together and I made an absolutely perfect landing. I'd finished my first solo flight! I was so pleased with myself that I completely failed to take any notice of the guy who was guiding me back to my parking space and managed to park with the wing of my plane underneath the wing of another plane. I then got hauled out of the cockpit by the other members of the flying club and summarily thrown fully-clothed into the swimming pool as my initiation into the ranks of the solo flyers.

As I was now a fully-fledged airman, Tommy Ellis built an airstrip at the back of the ranch, telling me it would be a great idea to put a plane back there. I wasn't so sure. It did seem a bit short and it was also surrounded by trees, but Tommy was convinced it would work. I still wasn't and because I reckoned I didn't have the experience to bring a plane in onto that strip I went back to the club and spoke to the manager and asked him if he would bring a plane over. He agreed and Tommy was delighted when the plane arrived.

He had got the champagne flowing copiously and he was in his element, constantly uttering one of his favourite sayings, "Soup for the boys!" He looked at the pilot, 'Now we'll take off together to celebrate.' The pilot looked at me and said it would be impossible as Tommy was too big and the plane would never get over the trees. Tommy was a difficult man to argue with so in desperation we sent him inside to organise some more drinks.

The pilot hopped in the plane and I quickly swung the prop for him as there was no electric starter. The trouble was, he had to taxi down to the end of the field to take off as the wind was wrong. The noise of the plane taxiing alerted Tommy, who came out of the house waving his fists and demanding to know what was happening. I told him he was just checking the field over for ruts at which point the plane turned into the wind and started to take off.

'Christ!' He yelled, 'The bastard's taking off' and he ran back inside only to reappear seconds later brandishing his elephant gun. He loosed off a shot but luckily he was so drunk that the kick from the massive weapon blew him straight onto his back whereupon we all leapt on him. No worries though, he'd already passed out and the plane and pilot escaped without any damage. You certainly didn't forget Tommy Ellis in a hurry.

I mentioned riding and this was something else I learned to do while out at the ranch. I had my own horse, called Zephyr. He was a wonderful animal and every time I went over to the stables and called his name his ears would prick up and he'd come cantering over to me. This probably had a lot to do with the pocketful of carrots I always carried as well but it's nice to think the feeling of affection was mutual.

I think I was a capable rider but as I've said many times before, I was a cocky so-and-so and would occasionally get my comeuppance. One such occasion happened on a cross country ride some friends and I went on to a well-known place called Half Way House. We'd been drinking and eating and of course were as happy as Larry and it probably goes without saying, not a little foolhardy.

'Come on, you guys,' I exhorted, as we were heading back to the ranch. 'There's only one way to show you're a true horseman and that is to cross your stirrups over your saddle, knot your reins, sit there with crossed arms and control the horse with your knees.'

'Well, you can bloody do it, we're not!' Came the eminently sensible reply.

So I did and was merrily trundling along, arms crossed and gripping with my knees, looking every inch the confident horseman. Everybody who's ever ridden knows that horses are often a little more urgent on the way back to their home and it was no different this time. As soon as they got the scent, they were off at full pelt. I hung on gamely with my knees until we hit the turn into the stables. Zephyr made the turn easily; I didn't and tried to go straight on. I'm still not sure how I managed to do it but as I flew from the saddle I somehow contrived to throw my legs around the horse's neck, just like a wrestling scissor-grip and hung on for dear life. Zephyr stopped dead and lowered me gently to the ground and as I lay there, his big brown eyes just looked down at me as if to say, "You bloody fool!"

Chapter 13
The Evil Within

For a poor Jewish kid from the East End, living in South Africa was wonderful. I had a horse to ride, a plane to fly and a maid to take care of me but of course, no chapter on living in South Africa at this time would be complete without mentioning apartheid.

When I arrived in South Africa in early 1948 the United Party were in power under Jan Smuts. After the second world war, Smuts had proposed the abolition of all segregation in the country. This, alongside his support for Britain during the war, had made him unpopular among the Afrikaner population and I remember working in the Stork Club, whose clientèle was largely British, when they announced Smuts had lost the 1948 general election to the segregationist National Party under Daniel Malan. Immediately a great depression fell over the club and nobody could enjoy themselves as we knew what it heralded. Before long, apartheid was enshrined in law and became a way of life.

Most musicians were not interested in politics or policies. The majority of people went about their business paying little or no attention to the fact that blacks had to use their own buses and toilets and that they had to have a pass to enter the city, which they had to vacate before dusk or heaven help them. It was effectively out of sight, out of mind to most people. They were denied education and if there were any black musicians, we never saw them. In any case, they wouldn't have been allowed to play in a white club. Myself, Herbie Kretzmer and Dave Lee weren't afraid to question what we saw and we called ourselves the Three Musketeers. This attitude would occasionally land us in trouble with the police and eventually the fallout from our continued non-acceptance would be one of the driving forces for leaving the country.

Ironically, the white South Africans loved jazz. Whether they were oblivious as to its origins or they accepted it as just being from another country, I don't know. I even remember Nat "King" Cole's "Nature Boy" being top of the hit parade over there for a while and being played on the radio all the time.

The government was determined to keep the blacks in the townships, such as Alexander Township. These were disgusting, ramshackle shanty-towns, devoid of sanitation, gas or electricity. Animals were kept in less cruel conditions. When we questioned people about the conditions all we'd get back was "well, would you want someone as filthy as that living next to you?" And when you countered by saying that if they had an education they could rise above the filth, you were labelled a communist. You couldn't argue with such ingrained bigotry.

The police were fearsome. They were almost all poorly educated Afrikaner "Yaapies" brought in to the city from the "dorps" or villages. While I was there, there was a story doing the rounds about the horse that had dropped dead on the corner of Bree and Von Weiligh Streets. Apparently the attending policeman dragged it to Bree because he couldn't spell Von Weiligh. However, supposed lack of intelligence or not, you crossed the police at your peril and they didn't need much of an excuse to create trouble when there were blacks involved. For intelligence, just substitute thuggery.

My cleaning lady was a lovely woman called Mary and she looked after me like a mother. I'd finish work at the club at 4am and sleep through until 11. While I was asleep she'd come in and quietly run a bath for me and then have breakfast ready for me by the time I was bathed and dressed. Then whenever I had a free night she would make a dinner party for my friends and I. I was in seventh heaven and I felt like a king. I never saw Mary as a second class citizen because as far as I was concerned she was employed as my home help, and an exceedingly fine one at that, doing her job as well as I did mine, probably even better. She was certainly not a slave.

Apartheid sadly forced me to view our relationship in a completely different way. Not that it changed the way I actually thought of Mary, of course, but she was black and as such she couldn't legally be anything but my servant and never my social equal. No way would I be publicly able to admit to a friendship, however platonic, with a black woman. To the government, the police, the church and much of the population, it was illegal, sinful and abhorrent to just be nice to a fellow human being.

One event brought home to me the futility of trying to act with any kind of humanity in a land ruled by inhuman thugs. Mary would cheerfully shop for all the food and do all the cooking and on one particular day she had bought too much food by mistake so I told her to take it home with her for her family. She left later on with two carrier bags full of food and a big smile across her face.

An hour after she left, I received a telephone call from the police to say that Mary had been arrested because she had been found in possession of two bags of food stolen from my home. I told them that it wasn't true; she hadn't stolen the food, I had given it to her and would they please give it back to her and let her go. They told me to stay in my home as they would be coming round to see me. When I opened the door a little later, two big Afrikaaner cops stormed in saying that if I gave any more things to the blacks they would give me 24 hours to leave the country. I protested that it wasn't a crime to give but they just replied that I was behaving like a communist and they would be watching me from their station and my name would be on their files.

It never took them long to decide what made someone a communist. The irony was, of course, is that I don't think they even understood what communism entailed. To them, calling someone a communist was more of an insult; an inherently "bad" thing to be and nothing to do with political dogma or ideology.

Dave Lee had a similar experience. He used to go to the local Bantu club to teach piano to the kids there. When the police found out about this they went and confronted him. They told him that they knew he was a communist, although not a very big one, and that if he told them who his superiors were he could stay, otherwise he would have 24 hours to leave the country. He obviously wasn't a communist and therefore had no superiors but as he couldn't produce any evidence of this, he had to go. Dave, who didn't hold a single political thought in his head, let alone a communist one, did manage to make a joke out of it though. He said that he wouldn't have minded so much if they'd called him a senior communist 'but to be labelled an insignificant one...'

Mary cried bitterly when I told her that I'd had enough of the system and was going to go back to England. She begged me to take her and her family with me and I would have done had I been able to but it was impossible for her, as a black, to leave the country. It seemed rather ironic that, given that they had had every other human right removed, they still had a nationality when it suited the government, and that this nationality was being used to deny them the remaining freedoms everyone else enjoyed. How Nelson Mandela kept his anger at bay for so many years and still managed to retain his dignity in the face of so much provocation and then finding the power of forgiveness is beyond me. He deserves a sainthood.

Many years later I would return to South Africa for a reunion with some the musicians I played with during those 5 years. This time the political regime was African, not Afrikaaner and I was stunned at the changes and the advances made towards racial equality. I was travelling on a courtesy bus coming back from Sun City and in the seat in front of me was an Afrikaaner guy sitting next to a black girl. He had his arm around her and was kissing her. I thanked God for the changes as even 20 years before they would both have been imprisoned. Or, heaven forbid, even worse.

Chapter 14
Coming Home

Were it not for the evil of apartheid, I would probably have stayed in South Africa like many of my old bandmates did. I couldn't though; I wasn't going to take the risk that my benevolence towards my fellow man could eventually land me in jail or at worst, even get me killed so I reluctantly made plans to return home to England. Going back to South Africa many years later and reuniting with many of my old friends still living and in many cases, still making music out there, made me realise what a marvellously full and interesting life I'd had since then. It's obvious to me now that I'm certain I made the right decision, however hard it may have seemed at the time. One thing I've always trusted is my instinct, whether it was for a deal or for making a potentially life-changing decision; something good has nearly always come from following it.

I was actually very excited by my return home. I'd accumulated so much baggage that I decided to return by ship and I caught the Union Castle in Durban after being given a big send-off by all my friends. The journey back was going to be two weeks with a few stops on the way. No way was I going to get bored!

It was very noticeable (and pleasant) that, after the ship left Cape Town where the overnight "bed and breakfast" passengers from Durban disembarked and the majority of the England-bound ones got on, we were no longer in South Africa and therefore no longer under the apartheid regime I hated so much. This was neatly illustrated one evening after I'd gone into one of the bars for a drink. There was an Afrikaaner at one of the tables who kept snapping his fingers impatiently at the waiter, trying to get his attention. The waiter deliberately ignored him but after it had gone on for a while, went over to him and told him, in a broad Cockney accent, "'ere, listen to me. You're not in Saarf Africa now, we're in international waters and I'm not one of yer Kaffir boys so you don't snap yer fingers at me. If you want me, you call 'steward' or my name, which is John. If you snap yer fingers, you'll be getting yer own drinks." Wonderful stuff and it put him neatly in his place.

The bandleader on board had heard I'd done some photography before so he asked me if I could help him out as he'd made a hash of the pictures he'd taken at the fancy dress balls and similar events on the outbound trip. I said it wouldn't be a problem and that I'd take care of it. Come the night of the fancy dress ball, I was the official ship's photographer. I was busily taking pictures of a dreary bunch of people when suddenly in walked a girl who, until then, we'd thought was very shy. Before, she'd always blushed and walked away whenever we talked to her. She certainly wasn't blushing tonight, her costume brought everything to a standstill; she was wearing an RAF jacket and cap, black lace stockings and suspenders and between her legs she'd placed the message "Target for Tonight". She posed happily and the ball came alive. Everyone wanted a copy of the picture and I was up all night printing them. The bandleader made quite a bit of money just from this one shot. He was very grateful but when he asked me what he owed me I said nothing - but I asked him whether he could loan me the use of his camera equipment when we got to Madeira, if that would be ok.

I'd heard of the famous Reid's Palace hotel in Funchal on Madeira. It was, and still is, one of those hotels like The Ritz or Raffles in Singapore where the atmosphere and service is second to none and people visit just to say they've been. It was too much of a temptation and I just had to try something out. I arrived at the hotel by taxi and immediately asked to see the manager. I explained that I was a photographer from National Geographic Magazine and that I'd been commissioned to take some pictures of the hotel kitchens. The manager was delighted and took me off to the kitchens where they were preparing the most fabulous food imaginable for lunch. I took some 'photographs' with my empty camera and asked him for some information about how the food was being prepared so I could put that in the article too; the lobster for instance...

"Perhaps sir would like to try it?"

How could I possibly resist? I sat down to a mouth-wateringly gorgeous lunch and afterwards I carried on round Madeira taking non-existent photographs and got my dinner as well! Maybe there was a little of my father's con-artist spirit still alive and kicking within me but I just prefer to think I've got a gift for sweet-talking. When I got back to the ship the bandleader said I could use his darkroom to develop the pictures but I said there was no need and told him what I'd been up to. He said he'd wished he'd been with me.

Leaving Madeira, the ship soon arrived back at Southampton and travelling back up to London on the boat train I began to feel depressed at the sight of all the houses bunched together with smoke belching from chimney pots into the cold leaden sky above. The contrast with the wide-open veldt and huge blue skies I'd been used to and taken so much for granted for the previous few years was immense.

The depression left me when I arrived at Waterloo Station and saw my father and my brother waiting there for me. The journey home to Forest Gate shot by as we talked non-stop all the way and that evening, all the relatives came round to the house to see me. I was now looking forward to regaling my eager audience with tales of my adventures from the far-flung reaches of the Empire and it seemed like we were in for a show as the front room had even been prepared for the event. After all the initial greetings, cups of tea and food, there was a loud 'Sshh! It's time, he's on!' No, it wasn't my cue: I hadn't noticed the tiny 12" television set in the corner of the room that was now flickering and crackling into life in order to show "What's My Line?" and its superstar panellist, the late Gilbert Harding. It would be another 20 years or so until television reached South Africa. What on earth had I come back to? So enthralled were my family by the television that nobody even noticed as I left the room and went into the kitchen to plan the next stage of my life.

-oo0oo-

While it was nice to be back, I was finding the restrictions of living back in the UK difficult to adjust to. For instance, if you wanted to travel you could only take £25 with you and how far would that go? My brother and some friends decided to go to Paris for a weekend and asked me along. We flew with BEA and hoped that our £25 each would cover the costs of our hotel and food. On our first night there we went in search of some night-life and ended up in a jazz club. The music was great and during the interval I asked the bass player if I could have a sit-in. When the band got back on the stage they made an announcement that there was a British bass player in the audience by the name of Tony Kaye who was invited to play the next set! There was a lot of applause and welcoming shouts as I got up to play the set and I took several solos and to my astonishment, received a standing ovation.

Sitting down afterwards the owner of the club came over and asked whether I would be interested in doing a similar guest spot every night while I was in Paris as it would be good for his business to have an English guest musician. When I asked him how much he would pay he said 1000 francs a night so we shook hands on the deal. It wasn't a fortune but at least we now had enough money to stay for a week, not just a weekend.

Returning to London, I started to wonder about what I was going to do now. I certainly wasn't going back into wrestling promotion and I really didn't fancy playing in a band again. Remembering the stuff I'd written and produced for the Sunday shows back in Margate, South Africa and the one I'd toured with in Germany while in the army, an idea started to germinate.

I began wondering if it was possible to take a show out to the American troops stationed in Germany. It was several years since my last visit and I had no idea how the procedures had changed so I went to see the agent who booked the shows for Germany, a gentleman by the name of Bert Wilcox, who said we would need to audition for him. If he thought it was OK we would then need to go to Frankfurt for a second audition in front of the USO (United Services Organization) board. Wages would be $30 per person per week if we passed the final audition.

After getting all the necessary information together I reckoned I could make it work, so I sat down and wrote a sophisticated little show. I'd selected musicians who could both play and clown around when needed to and also three girls who could sing, dance and act. The arrangements were all written by Bernard Ebbinghouse, who would later go on to become a renowned composer and arranger for film and TV. We rehearsed and then went and auditioned for the London agent, who thought we were great. He phoned the USO in Frankfurt and he told us to come over. At this time I was financing everything with my savings so what with the wages I was paying everyone and the cost of the fares to Germany it meant my money was running out fast. We'd better get the job otherwise I would be broke. Not only broke but stranded in Germany and broke!

When we got to Frankfurt we watched all the other shows audition and we thought we would walk it as they were all so corny. Imagine our disappointment when, after we'd finished our audition, a major in the USO came over and said that he was very sorry but they couldn't use us as it wasn't the right kind of material for the troops.

I was dumbfounded. I thought we were so sophisticated and that that would be enough. Unfortunately that wasn't what the soldiers wanted; they preferred slapstick clowning around, Spike Jones type stuff. I didn't know what to do and I was rather overcome with the shock of realising I didn't have enough money left to get everyone back to the UK after I'd used every last penny to produce the show. I asked whether the USO could give me another week to do a re-write and then do another audition and to my immense relief, they agreed and they even provided our hotel accommodation and food. Now all I needed to do was write a good, slick show and have it all rehearsed and ready in the space of one week.

I knew now that they wanted corny and slapstick so it wasn't too difficult putting the show together. I wrote for a couple of days then we rehearsed it and by the end of the week we had a show to audition. It included a drunken skit of "Zing Went The Strings Of My Heart" and corny dance routines and quite frankly, we were embarrassed doing it. I coerced and cajoled the troupe by saying it was money for old rope and to stick with it. We were last on at the audition and at the end of our spot the same USO major as before came over and booked us, The Tony Kaye Band, for a lengthy tour of US military bases. The USO in Germany paid us $30 per person per week in scrip, a form of credit currency. There were hotels in Germany subsidised by the US government and we'd pay the scrip equivalent of 50c per day for a room, bed, breakfast and lunch. Our evening meals would usually be provided by the venue. The balance of our money would then be converted and paid to us when we returned to England.

Again, a dreadful admission but my memory is so awful now that I can't remember anyone's name from my own band. I hope no-one is offended but if you're reading this, I'm sorry! One name I do remember though is that of the brilliant alto-sax player Joe Harriott. He went on to become an inspirational player to many but he never made it past rehearsals for the Tony Kaye Band because he refused to do the comedy stuff.

While on tour, I noticed that there was a genuine need for quality musicians to accompany the touring artistes so I approached the USO agent in Germany, a Belgian named Albert Licart, and offered to supply them. So now I had a foot in the door with agency work and things were looking up very nicely.

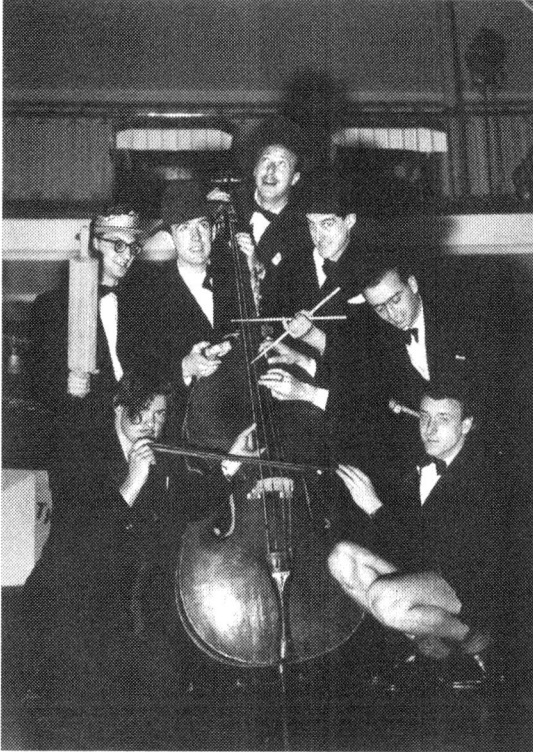

The Tony Kaye Band as we were in Germany

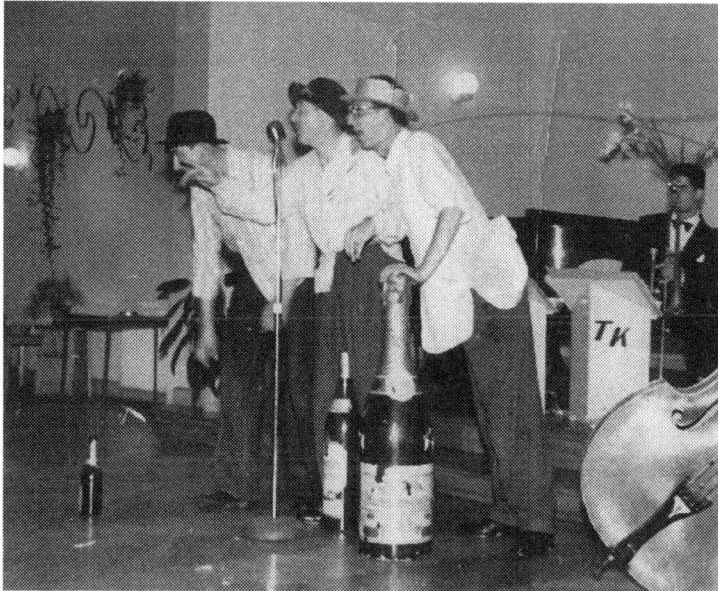

Pleasing the troops

Back home in Britain I carried on with the agency work with differing success. Ironically, Teddy Foster came to me and asked if I could get him any work. The music scene was changing and work for big bands was becoming difficult to get but I told him that there was a possibility with Granada on their cine-variety bills. Teddy thought it was worth a try so I made an appointment to see they guy who was in charge of cine-variety at Granada. When I arrived, his secretary apologised saying that he had had to go off to a meeting suddenly but that I could go over everything with her.

Her name was Lillian. I offered to take her out to lunch and she agreed. Over our meal I realised that we were talking about everything except the Teddy Foster Band so when I met Teddy later and he asked me if I'd got anywhere, I had to say that I didn't think I had but that I thought I'd met my future wife.

In 1954 I got a booking for the Tony Kaye Band to play at the US Mission to Luxembourg, at a ball for the appointment of the new Minister, Wiley T. Buchanan (he would later be the first Ambassador to the Grand Duchy). My pal from South Africa, Dick Norton was now working at Radio Luxembourg and had become friendly with the people at the American Mission. They had asked him to find a band from the UK to play at the ball so he contacted me. The previous Minister, who was also attending, was none other than Perle Mesta. She was a legendary socialite, the original "Hostess with the Mostest" and was the subject of the Irving Berlin musical "Call Me Madam" starring Ethel Merman. When I asked which music we should play at the booking I was told in no uncertain terms that numbers from "Call Me Madam" were definitely not to be on the bill! We made the news at home, too. One of the music papers of the time, I think it was the Melody Maker, featured a headline along the lines of "First British Band to Play Luxembourg". Fame at last!

Immediately after the ball I met up with Dick Norton, who took me back to the studios to make his regular broadcast to London and during it he allowed me to send a short message to my future wife.

Then after the radio show I headed off to Frankfurt to meet Albert Licart in order to collect the money he owed me for my artists. It was lucky that I'd chosen that day to go as any later and I would have left a lot of people out of pocket. When I arrived at his office his secretary told me that I wouldn't be able to see him as he was in a meeting. I looked around the reception area and something didn't seem right. It was a bit too empty for my liking so I ignored the secretary and went into Licart's office. Again, it looked suspiciously empty, except for Licart, who was in the middle of cleaning out the contents of his safe. It was like a scene from a B-movie and he was, it's reasonable to say, astonished to see me. He was quite obviously about to do a runner with all the money he was meant to be paying me and several other acts he handled. I made him hand over the money he owed me there and then. Regrettably I couldn't do anything about the money he owed the other shows as I didn't know who they were and I can only hope that somehow they caught up with him too.

I saw a chance to maybe capitalise on this as there would obviously be an agent's license available and that would suit me down to the ground. I complained to the USO person in charge of entertainment who said he couldn't do anything to stop him and that any complaint could only be brought by the acts he represented. He did say that if it were true and he was swindling the acts, he would remove his USO agent's licence. I asked him there and then whether he would consider giving me his licence if he was found to be a crook. He refused and gave no reason. I later found out that he was anti-semitic so he certainly wasn't going to be doing me any favours.

Chapter 15
Hair

Not getting the USO agency licence was a knock-back I didn't really need and was the nail in the coffin of my ambitions to become a successful agent. I was now also engaged to be married and would shortly need the extra finance that entailed. Yet again, I was at a loss as to what I could do for a career and needed that spark of inspiration. My mother provided it this time by bizarrely suggesting I take up hairdressing. Hairdressing was the furthest thing from my mind as a career – I was 28 for heaven's sake and she expected me to learn how to cut hair? Never.

I still used to visit the Archer Street musicians' hang-outs and just down the road from Archer Street, on the corner of Shaftsbury Avenue and Piccadilly Circus, was the well-known Morris School of Hairdressing. I'd passed this so many times before and never given it a second thought but one day, prompted by Mother's suggestion, I walked up to see what was going on. I chatted to the people there and before I knew it, I'd signed up for a six-month hairdressing course. It was a spur of the moment decision that would change my life.

The first day I walked into the training school there was a group of kids all sat around in a circle learning how to do pin curls and I was expected to join straight in! I looked across the room and blow me down I recognised the face opposite. It belonged to a tenor sax player I knew.

'What are you doing here?' I asked

'I was going to ask you the same question.'

He told me he'd been playing with Ray Noble in New York but had come back because he wanted to do something outside of music. After one week at the school I began to get the hang of this hairdressing lark. Unfortunately he didn't, decided to quit the course and went back to music.

By the time the six months were up, I'd become friends with Alfred Morris and his wife. They even joined my fiancée and me in a box at the Chelsea Arts Club New Year's Eve ball at the Royal Albert Hall in 1954. This was one of the "in" events for New Year's Eve and Lillian's brother had the photography concession. It was a boisterous affair; fancy dress, as always, with live music. Traditionally there was a parade of models that had been prepared by students and this year one group had painted nude models in gold and these were being chased by another group of students with paint remover! Everyone had had a bit too much to drink by the time it finished around 4am but it was great fun and there was no trouble.

Alfred introduced me to John Oates. He'd been a stylist with Raymond Bessone, better known as television's "Mr Teasy Weasy" but he now ran his own salon in Dublin. He offered me a job working for him there and I thought it would be a good idea to accept. Although I'd proved to be quite a good hairdresser, I thought it would be a good move to go and refine my craft in an out of the way place like Dublin where nobody knew me. I'd be able to learn a lot from someone like John and then hopefully move back to London a while later as the finished product. But first I had another matter to attend to and Lillian and I got married on May 30th, 1955. We immediately went off to live in the Ballsbridge area of Dublin.

John Oates had a very nice salon opposite the famous Gaiety Theatre in Dublin and had built up an excellent clientèle. I did indeed learn a lot from both John and Joan, his wife. I began to develop my own clientèle too, which was a very reassuring testament to my burgeoning skills as a stylist. One day a lady came in for an appointment and I did the booking. While she was sitting under the dryer having her hair set and unable to hear us talking, John came over to me and asked whether I had any idea who she was. When I said I didn't, he told me that she was Sybil Connelly's sister. I had to apologise because I was still none the wiser. John explained that Sybil Connelly was a top fashion designer and that she did lots of work in America, especially California. She always sent her sister in whenever there was a new hairdresser so that she could try him out. If she liked what she saw, she would come in herself. She would be a very important feather in my cap so I did the best I could.

Naturally I was now rather nervous. This was my first high-profile client but I remained confident, combed her hair out and finished her off. All she said was thank you and after giving me a tip, she left. Ten minutes went by and the telephone rang. John answered it, had a brief conversation with the caller and then came back to me and said, 'You've done it! She's just made an appointment!' She turned out to be a charming client and we got on very well. She must have been quite impressed with me because she offered me a position as her resident hairdresser for all her shows. I didn't accept but it was nice to be thought of all of a sudden as a major force in the Dublin hairdressing culture.

After several months learning the ropes in Dublin we were ready to move back to London and take on the challenge of working there. Our first home was in the unused basement of my in-laws' house in Kensington that my Uncle Syd and I had converted into a flat. It was our new home but it signalled the end of part of my old life. One evening I invited some of my old musician friends round and we spent a great time reminiscing over drinks. My wife detested them and said she never wanted them in the house again. I have sadly lost touch with many of them over the years as we went our different ways. It's terrible to have a door closed on part of your life that way but as ever, when one door closes, another often opens.

The owners of the well-known Martin Douglas René chain of salons, the Webb family, were friends and neighbours of my family from Forest Gate, so I went and paid them a visit. Their main salon was next door to Claridges Hotel in Davis Street, Mayfair but they also had salons in many of the department stores. Their clientèle was a quality one; very top-drawer with many society ladies, top models and film stars. Although they were called Martin Douglas René, René had left by this time. He was very popular among society ladies and one of René's clients was Princess Margaret. They had a vacancy for the position of manager in the salon at Penberthy's department store in Oxford Street. I felt very lucky to get offered this chance so early on in my career so I took it.

The salon didn't have a lot of custom when I took it over so being the manager it was up to me to think of ways of building up the business. I had some fliers printed up and distributed to all the offices in the area. These were aimed at all the female office staff and invited them for cheese and wine along with a free styling and colouring consultation. There weren't many invitations like this in 1956 and we were mobbed. I even had to take on extra staff such was the success of my little initiative! Of course, we think nothing of that kind of PR today and invitations like that often end up in the bin. Half a century ago it was a relatively novel approach and I've always been willing to try something new. Innovation alongside the zeal of the old market trader proved to be a winning combination on many occasions throughout my career.

I stayed at Penberthy's for a couple of years but was once again starting to feel I wasn't going anywhere. We had a surprise visit from my sister-in-law who lived in Stanford, Connecticut and she suggested I was wasting my talent in London and why didn't I go to America where I could earn more money and work in better salons? I talked it over with Lillian, we decided she'd had a point and that we would go. My wife went out first, staying with her sister while I was left to sell up our small home and work out my notice with the salon. I was travelling again.

Chapter 16
New York, New York

When we arrived in the States I found out that one had to have a licence to work as a hairstylist and that this entailed first spending six months in a hairdressing school. I didn't have enough money to keep us for six months so I took a chance and went along to the hairdressing school, showed them my diplomas from London and said I could teach their teachers! To my good fortune they agreed and they gave me a licence to work in the State of New York.

My first job didn't last long. It was in the world-famous Waldorf Astoria Hotel of all places and I was very excited at going to work in such a prestigious location. Until, that is, I walked in to the salon. It was like the dark ages; there were curtained cubicles in which almost everything was done. The manageress told me that my first client was in cubicle three and just as I was about to draw back the curtain to the cubicle I heard a deep masculine voice from within. My God, I thought, my first client was a man – surely not? I hadn't been trained with men's hair, I was a ladies' stylist, not a barber. I pulled back the curtain to see a plump woman being given a manicure and it was her voice I had heard, talking to the manicurist. She turned to me: "You're the Englishman; they always give me any new stylists because I'm a very difficult client. Now, young man, this is how I want you to set my hair…" Too pompous by half and I took an instant dislike to her.

"Madam, you are right, I am the Englishman. My status is that of a hairstylist which means I am an artist in my own right and you, madam, are insulting me by telling me how to set your hair in order to get the result you desire. Either I set your hair my way or you can get someone else to do it!" At that she screamed for the manager and insisted I be fired on the spot. I didn't bother to wait for the manager and walked out, relieved, because there was no way I could have worked in such a terrible environment. A more inauspicious start to my career in the USA I couldn't have made.

The next job was better and far more satisfying. I worked for a guy named Eddie Senz who was the head of make up for NBC TV studios (his brother was a famous wig-maker who made rugs for such luminaries as Bing Crosby and Rex Harrison). Eddie and I would travel to the studios and he would do make-up and I would style. I did hair for quite a few well-known clients but I remember two for quite different reasons. I once did the actress Virginia Gilmore's hair and shared a taxi with her. She offered to pay but I wouldn't have anything of it. After she got out, the cab-driver turned round to me and asked if I was crazy. "That was Yul Brynner's wife – she's loaded!"

The second was the beautiful but ultimately tragic Jean Seberg. I had been roused early one morning to do her hair and she was very gracious about inconveniencing me. I still have a signed picture of her that she gave to me. On the back of it she had written, "Anthony, forgive me for getting you up on a Monday morning. Next time let's both hope it's in the evening and in a theater." I never did make that date and after being hounded by the FBI for her support of radical causes throughout the 1970s, all the while alongside an increasingly complex personal life, she took her life in 1979. A very sad end for a wonderful talent.

The top hairdresser in New York at the time was Enrico Caruso and I was lucky enough to be hired by him. I did some studio work with him for Revlon and Clairol, which I found very interesting but he also dealt with a very select clientèle and had a salon at the Round Hill Hotel in Montego Bay, Jamaica. My wife and I were experiencing a few problems and I wanted to get away for a while so I asked Enrico whether I could go to Jamaica and manage the salon there. Initially he refused but after I explained why I wanted to go, he agreed. I packed my bags and set off to Jamaica for three and a half of the most wonderful months of my life.

To say that Enrico's clients were different class was not an exaggeration. They were drawn from all levels of what could be termed American society. Whereas British society was based on your birthright, American society was built around the twin pillars of wealth and celebrity. Jamaica, by virtue of it being beyond the pocket of the average man in the street, was one of the places the rich and famous went to unwind away from the public gaze. Nowadays the media has the power to make celebrities of almost anyone but the ones I found myself mixing with here were superstars, many of them global ones. I looked one way and I'd be staring at Bing Crosby; turn around and I'd bump into Oscar Hammerstein or Ethel Merman. What was even nicer was that I was doing all the ladies' hair, celebrity or wife thereof, and making friends with all of them. I had an immense amount of fun.

-oo0oo-

I had a nickname in the salon there; I was known as "The Cantankerous Englishman". Unfortunately although I'm a patient man, a certain kind of fool is very difficult to suffer gladly and wealthy ladies in hairdressing salons can sometimes lead the field among these. I got the name after dealing with one such woman who demanded that I put "pink rollers here, blue rollers there, curls here, that there" alongside sundry other demands. I was becoming increasingly frustrated until I snapped, picked up a tray that had rollers, clips and a razor on and put it down on her lap.

"What's this?" she demanded.

"A do it yourself kit" I replied and walked away.

She went running into the manager's office screaming that I'd given her a razor to cut her throat with. John, the manager, who knew her and her antics well simply told her, "That's Anthony for you."

From doing his wife's hair I'd become friendly with Oscar Hammerstein, the lyricist. He was a most delightful man and not at all the big star he was entitled to be. This was the man who had written the lyrics for some of the biggest stage and screen shows of all time such as Showboat, Oklahoma! and South Pacific; who was a double Oscar winner (the only person named Oscar to win one) and here I was having a couple of quiet drinks with him on the terrace of a posh hotel in Jamaica. A cruise ship had just docked and disgorged her passengers for a shore excursion. Now, the terrace didn't have air-conditioning; instead it had louvred windows that picked up the trade winds. The first passenger from the cruise ship arrived, an archetypal American tourist of that era with the Hawaiian shirt, baseball cap, cigar and obligatory two cameras slung round his fat neck. As he walked in the first thing he said was, "Jeez! Ain't they got no air conditioning in dis joint?" At which point Oscar slid down in his chair muttering to me, "Now you know why they wrote "The Ugly American"." (A bestseller at the time by William J. Lederer and Eugene Burdick).

Another time I was in the salon and a woman came in asking me to give her bangs. This wasn't a proposition, it's what we'd call a fringe in the UK. I suggested to her that if she really wanted to look like Shirley Temple then she should go elsewhere. She told me that that was the way she always wore her hair and that she wasn't changing now. I then told her that she ought to look like the elegant woman she undoubtedly was and not like the child she most certainly wasn't. At which she relented and let me have my head. And I did. Afterwards, she signed the bill but also gave me an amazing $100 tip, a huge amount of money back then. After about half an hour a man came into the salon. He was dressed all in white; cap, shirt, socks, everything and was smoking a big cigar. He demanded to speak to the guy who set his wife's hair. As I was the only man in the place it had to be me he was after. I nervously asked him what the problem was.

"Young man, I wanna shake you by the hand. You're the first guy who's had the balls to tell my wife what to do. My name's Crown, Colonel Crown. Whenever you come to Chicago, I'll build you the best salon you've ever seen."

The name meant nothing to me but I thanked him anyway and said I'd certainly consider his most generous offer (although I needed a salon in Chicago like I needed a hole in the head). We used to get a VIP list every day to tell us who was in and right at the top of the list was Colonel Crown, which more or less indicated he was indeed pretty important. It transpired that not only did he own about half of Chicago, he also owned New York's Empire State Building (which he would sell in a year or so in one of the biggest real estate deals ever seen). Maybe I should have taken him up after all!

Yet another offer came from another hugely wealthy man, Winthrop Rockefeller. Winthrop and his wife asked me to go to Puerto Rico for them. They'd opened a hotel there and they wanted me to run the salon, right away - they'd fly me out immediately! I said I couldn't just leave and close the Jamaica salon as Enrico would lose money. No problem, they would reimburse Enrico; they really were determined but so was I - to stay. It became quite a battle to convince them that I couldn't go but they backed down in the end. Winthrop was quite a character; he used to come into the bar, sit on a stool and drink until he fell off it. Then he used to call up to the barman, "John, serve me down here!" In a few years he would be elected Governor of Arkansas and oversee the introduction of pioneering race-relations legislation. His charitable foundation would also give away millions of dollars to a legion of worthwhile causes.

Having access to all these wealthy ladies and their husbands, and moreover being trusted by them, meant I could also act as a kind of middle man. A retired ballet dancer who had given up dancing after an injury to his back, came in one day and asked me a favour. He was now a portrait painter and was looking for new clients. He told me that if I could secure him a commission, there would be something in it for me. I didn't want to recommend anything blind so I asked to see his portfolio. The next day he came in with some wonderful pictures so I said I'd try and help him out. That same day, Charlotte Ford, daughter of Henry, came in for an appointment so I just happened to show her the pictures. She thought they were great too and asked me to fix up a meeting. She ended up having her portrait done and was so impressed she asked him to do her father as well. Later I heard he was about to do Jackie Kennedy when JFK was assassinated.

Of course, being in a resort hotel, music and musicians were never far away and one time, temptation (and rum punch) got the better of me. The American entertainer Pat Boone was staying and his wife had been in to the salon in the morning to have her hair done. My boss Enrico, and his wife, were also down for the week and they invited me to dinner. We finished the meal and were having coffee out in the open when it started to rain unexpectedly. Rain was a pretty rare occurrence there and usually if it happened during the day, everyone would dash inside to the bar, where an impromptu rum punch party would often be held that would knock everyone out until evening. This time, as it was already evening, we just went into the bar for a few more drinks. Also inside was a small rostrum where a little jazz group was playing.

I was sufficiently lubricated by this point to sidle up to the bass player and ask him if I could have a sit-in. He was used to lots of people asking this but the usual request was to play drums.

"Man, drummer don't let his skins out to anyone!"

"No, I don't want to play drums, I want to play bass."

"Man, you got it!"

And he stuck the bass in my hand. For a moment I didn't know what to do with the instrument, I was paralysed. Then the pianist turned round and very disdainfully instructed me that for my information, we were in B flat. That was enough, I started to play. Suddenly the drummer said, "Hey this white cat's cool – give him four bars." They gave me four and the drummer took another four and slowly everyone stopped playing until it was just myself and the drummer left, trading licks. We were really swinging and by now the talking had stopped in the bar. Then Pat Boone came over, sat in the crook of the bass and said to me, "As a hairdresser you're a mean bass player, let's form a trio and go on tour!" The managing director came over and joked that we ought to do it every week. That was until I showed him my fingers; I told him he could either have a hairdresser or a bass player but not both as I'd got a bit carried away and had blisters on my fingers the size of acorns!

The three and a half months I spent in Jamaica were a truly wonderful time. I'd known nobody when I'd arrived but when I left I had a send off party at the airport with about 20 people all bearing gifts. It was very touching. I'd learned a lot there too. I'd been managing a successful salon with a high profile clientèle, experience I would be able to draw on in the future. That future was, for the time being, back in England.

Chapter 17
All at Sea

I've made a conscious decision not to go into too much detail about either of my marriages in this book. As far as I was concerned, I entered into both marriages with the right intentions but they both failed and I don't really want, or indeed need, to go over the reasons why. Necessity means I have had to refer to a few things here and there but there isn't any requirement to go into specific detail. That being said, incidents happened that had direct influence on our finances, where we lived and even why certain decisions were made and by not mentioning them there are a few obvious gaps. I hope the reader understands my reasons for wanting these details kept private. I could fill several chapters with the intricacies surrounding two failed marriages but this book is about me and I'm determined it shall stay that way.

-oo0oo-

When we came back to England we needed a place to stay while Lillian and I tried to calm some of the turbulence in our marriage. Tiny Webb, the eldest of the Webb brothers, owners of Martin Douglas René, suggested we stay with them in Bournemouth. I had managed to save some money in the US and I was planning to open my own salon back in England with it if I couldn't find the right job. Unfortunately the money didn't last long so I had to find a job. I went up to London to meet with my old employers at Martin Douglas René and thankfully they offered me a position back at their main salon in Davis Street.

Oddly enough, there was a chance I could have yet again gone back into music. While in town I took the opportunity to catch up with a few old friends. We went to the Kenya Coffee House in Marylebone High Street and who should walk in while we were sitting there but the bandleader Joe Loss. Our paths hadn't crossed for almost a decade and a half and although I'd never actually worked with him, we had known each other. Immediately he saw me he told me that he was just about to go on tour but that he was a bass player down. Would I like to join him? When I told him that I'd given up music for hairdressing he took one look at me and told me he didn't believe it!

Joe cropped up again many years later, this time in a much more indirect, yet still surprising manner. When I first saw my present flat a few years ago it was a little like stepping back into the 50s. It was a touch shabby here and there but I felt strangely drawn to it all the same, so I bought it. I spent a few quid doing it up nicely and I actually had the Times do a lifestyle feature on it, complete with a picture. When they published it there were quite a few enquiries from people and the paper passed these on to me. One of them turned out to be from a woman who said that her mother had been the previous occupant and that her mother was in fact Joe Loss' sister in law. Had I been receptive to some hidden "vibration" in the fabric of the flat? I'll never know.

Once again I was finding myself in contact with some high profile clients as I dealt with some of the gentry and quite a few stars as well. The late Diana Dors and Ingrid Bergman were both clients of the salon, as was a young Susan Hampshire. Unlike in Jamaica, we never got to socialise with the customers. Obviously one was able to talk and laugh with them during their appointments but it was very much an upstairs/downstairs relationship and fraternisation was definitely out of the question. There was one little secret we were party to: some of the blonde glamour girls who used to come in wanted to appear "natural" blondes, so they would take advantage of our tinting room to "complete" the look. I'm not talking about the hair on their heads either. The company also put me in charge of the school of hairdressing they had started up at the rear of the salon. I became very busy indeed.

I was there for a couple of years. It was a hard job and it left little time for the hands on business of styling. I was working long hours as not only was I running the school and teaching, I was also overseeing all the outside salons around the UK; checking their orders and taking care of their day-to-day problems. It was like running your own business but not really being in charge. There was the same amount of hassle and stress involved but without the reward.

Some of the clients used to come into the salon and talk about the cruises they'd been on. They used to say that everything was wonderful except for the onboard salons and this started me thinking. If I was working all hours God sends and wearing myself out just for a salary and no recognition, why not do the same and be my own boss? I started making enquiries about getting into the cruise business but didn't really have a clue who to ask.

One of my brothers-in-law was a photographer with concessions on cruise liners so I asked him about any possible openings with the companies he was working for. He said there was a company called Greek Line who operated from Greece to New York and they had just bought a ship from Netherland Line. They were going to rename and refit it and operate it out of Southampton running cruises to Madeira and the Canary Islands. It had a basic salon on board so why didn't I approach them and ask about the concession? It seemed the perfect opportunity so I arranged an interview and amazingly, considering I was completely new to the cruise market, I was given the contract. I hadn't even had time to form a company, instead I presented myself as "Anthony Kaye, trading as Coiffeur Transocean".

I went down to Southampton, had a look at the salon and decided it needed tarting up a bit to make it look more professional and up-to-date. So I spent what little money I had saved doing that and then I got a few staff together to man the salon, including one or two from

Martin Douglas René, and we were up and running. The new company, Coiffeur Transocean, was eventually incorporated in March 1963 and everything I now had was concentrated on this exciting new venture; on board the TSMS Lakonia. I wasn't to know it at the time but the next couple of years would either be the making or breaking of me.

Chapter 18
Tragedy

It all started very well. The cruises out of Southampton to the Canaries proved popular and business was picking up. Holiday cruising was still a huge novelty in the early '60s but there were new lines starting up all the time, not only in the UK but also all over Europe, so it was becoming much more affordable. It gave a lot of decent ordinary people a little touch of the high-life they'd read about in magazines or seen in the movies. The Lakonia was also one the grand old ladies of the sea and offered a little glimpse of the glories of pre- and post-war shipboard life. She originally went into service as a liner with Netherland Line in 1930 as the Johan van Oldenbarneveld and had also done stirling work as a troop ship during the war, earning the nickname "The Lucky Ship" as she was adept at avoiding attack. Post war service saw her operating as a round-the-world cruiser and also sailing to Australia and New Zealand. She was an immensely popular ship with all who sailed on her. Greek Line bought her in early 1963 and had her refitted in Genoa before she went into service as the Lakonia.

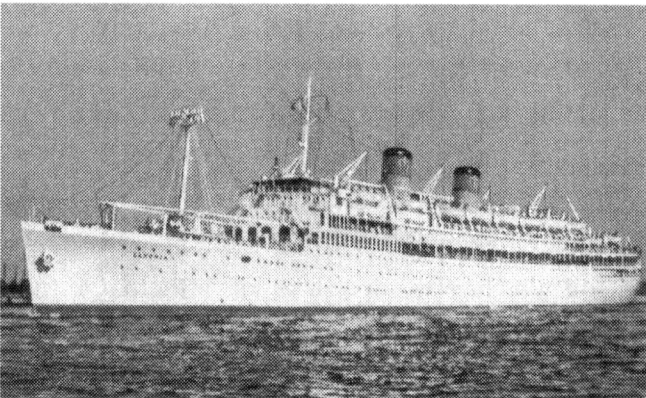

TSMS Lakonia. A Greek Line postcard of the grand old lady.

I soon realised though that to be able to make a decent living I would need to expand. A one-ship operation would never be enough so I went in search of more contracts. Attracted by my background with Martin Douglas René, the Royal Mail Steam Packet Company offered me one on their ship the Andes, a very upmarket vessel, as were all of the Royal Mail ships. They sent me a letter of intent and I started to celebrate. Then Royal Mail came back to me and asked me more about Martin Douglas René and it was only then I explained that there appeared to have been a misunderstanding as I was no longer with them. At which point they got cold feet and pulled out of the deal.

My solicitor said that as I had received a letter of intent I had grounds to sue as what they'd done constituted a broken contract. Where many would have sued, I decided not to. I was determined that my future was going to be in this industry and I didn't want to jeopardise it by getting a name as a trouble maker just as I was starting out. It was a relatively small industry back then and it wouldn't take long for gossip and rumour to spread round it. I telephoned Royal Mail and told them I respected their decision and that I wouldn't be holding them to their letter of intent but that I would appreciate it if they could cover my expenses, which they duly did.

My next chance came with a company called Typaldos who were arranging a Christmas cruise around the Greek islands on the Akropolis (whose identical sister ship, the Athinai would later feature as the "body double" for the star in Lew Grade's cult flop movie, "Raise The Titanic"). I couldn't afford to send staff out just for two weeks so I decided to go and do both the gents and ladies hairdressing all by myself. My staff were by now an experienced team well capable of handling the Lakonia's own Christmas cruise without my supervision so I was happy enough to leave them. On the evening of 19th December, Captain Mathios Zarbis slipped his command from her berth between the two grand Cunard Queens, Elizabeth and Mary at

Southampton en route the Canary Islands, for what would prove to be an unforgettable cruise for the 1022 passengers and crew on board.

It's unusual how tiny, seemingly insignificant details can sometimes stick in the memory because of their association with something rather more memorable. On the 23rd December 1963 I was busy in the barbershop attending to a gentleman who had very tight and curly hair when the radio officer hurried in. He was carrying a message for me and as he passed it across he warned me that it contained bad news. I expected possibly a death in the family and as I nervously opened the envelope I saw that the message was from my wife in London. It was a long one and was very bad news indeed.

She said the Lakonia had caught fire and that my team was being blamed for it. The press were now banging on the door and asking for statements and could I get home as soon as possible. I couldn't believe the news but I still had a job to do as the chap with the curly hair was still sitting in the chair. In shock, I took a large chunk of the poor gentleman's hair out without thinking, although I managed to talk him into having a crew-cut. He left looking like one of the first skinheads and after that cruise ended, I never cut hair again. I was unable to leave the Akropolis until the end of the cruise in Pireaus, two days away; two days of worry and two days before I could get anywhere near the facts about what had happened.

A few days prior to the ill-fated cruise, the Lakonia had undergone a quick re-fit and some engine modifications in Southampton as she had been losing speed on her recent sailings. She had passed a Ministry of Transport safety inspection the day before sailing and she left, only a few hours later than planned, on the 19th December. The first three days went by without incident. Around 11pm on the evening of the 22nd December the ship was still 180 miles north of its first port of call in Madeira and most of the passengers were enjoying the "Tropical Tramps" Ball in the Lakonia room, the ship's ballroom. Meanwhile a steward was passing the hairdressing salon and saw thick black smoke seeping under the door and on opening it, he found the salon completely ablaze. The fire burst out into the corridor but the steward, by now accompanied by another crewmember attempted to fight the blaze with extinguishers. Realising it was a hopeless task one of them ran off to alert the purser.

The passengers in the Lakonia Room had noticed the smell but not thought anything of it, believing it to be strong cigar smoke, and carried on dancing. When he was informed of the unfolding drama, Captain Zarbis went to the bridge and attempted to make an intercom announcement but the system had been rendered inactive by the fire. On top of that, the fire alarm was almost inaudible. Smoke soon began filling the ballroom though and the cruise director, George Herbert, took charge and marshalled the by now frightened passengers towards the boat deck. The wireless operator, Antonios Kalogridis, sent out the first distress call at 11.30pm. He sent the final call at 12.22am, shortly before the radio room succumbed to the blaze: "SOS from Lakonia, last time. I cannot stay anymore in the wireless station. We are leaving the ship. Please immediate assistance. Please help." The pressure boilers began to explode causing black smoke to spread throughout the ship and the order to abandon ship was given by the purser a little before 1am. Kalogridis was later seen leaving the ship in a launch accompanied by two musicians and a nurse although he maintained that he was actually actively involved in searching for survivors, not fleeing. This kind of accusation would later be rife.

The fire had taken hold very quickly and there was no way the six-man fire crew was able to contain it. A week before sailing the crew had taken part in a boat drill and the day after departure the passengers also undertook one to familiarise themselves with the evacuation procedure. It wasn't to be of much use and it later became obvious that not all the boats had been used in the safety drills. Despite the ship passing the safety inspection prior to leaving Southampton and holding a Greek certificate of seaworthiness, many of the lifeboats failed to lower properly as the winch mechanisms and chains on some of the davits were rusted. Boats stuck as they were lowered, one dangled precariously from one end, tipping its precious cargo into the sea and a davit broke as another boat was being lowered. Other lifeboats became swamped in the water as some of the drain holes weren't plugged so passengers had to continually bail water; other boats were burnt in the fire. In fact, it later transpired that only 5 lifeboats had been fully lowered in the crew's drill. Lockers containing lifejackets and safety equipment were impossible to open and some of the crew were mistakenly accused of looting staterooms when in fact they were searching for spare lifejackets.

There was a confusing mixture of orderliness and panic; ropes and ladders were lowered but a few passengers couldn't wait and jumped overboard. Some of them hit the side of the ship on the way down and were dead before they hit the water. Others headed for the stern area where the enclosed Agora shopping area was located and remained there for a few hours before the fire reached them. When it did, they lowered ladders and gangways and just walked into the sea, escaping to the liferafts that had been dropped by the rescue vessels that soon arrived on the scene.

The first ship to arrive around 3.30am was the Argentinian liner, Salta. She was soon joined by the British tanker Montcalm and between them they picked up most of the survivors. Several other vessels as well as four American C-54 rescue planes from the Azores joined in the search. These dropped life rafts and other survival gear and were able to spot passengers in the water. The main problem was that the ship was drifting and survivors and bodies were spread over several square miles of sea. Fortunately the water was warm and this along with the large number of search vessels ensured that casualties were minimised.

In traditional manner, the last person to leave the burning ship was Captain Zarbis, who was spotted walking around on deck shortly after daybreak and was rescued by a lifeboat from the Belgian vessel Charlesville. My manageress, Debbie Gould, was pictured in one of the national newspapers being rescued after spending ten hours in the sea. Despite the warm water it's still a wonder she managed to survive that long. All in all, 95 passengers and 33 crew died or were listed as missing. Only 53 were actually casualties of the fire itself and many of those bodies were recovered by crewmen of the British aircraft carrier, HMS Centaur. The rest of the fatalities were either through drowning, exposure or from injuries received from diving overboard. It was, at the time, one of the largest post-war peace-time maritime tragedies and should never have happened.

The Lakonia paid the ultimate price, too. The Norwegian tug, Herkules got a line aboard and with the aid of three other tugs began to tow her to Gibraltar. At 2pm on the 29th December, the day before the liner was due to return to Southampton, she developed an alarming list, keeled over on to her right hand side and within three minutes had sunk 1200 fathoms to the bottom of the Atlantic. By some tragic coincidence, she now lay on the bottom not too far from where her sister ship, the Marnix van St. Aldegonde, rested. She had been torpedoed and sunk by the Germans while acting as a troopship during WWII.

The aftermath of the disaster was terrible. I arrived back in Pireaus at the offices of Greek Line to all sorts of accusations arising from the fact that the fire had first been seen emanating from the salon. In almost everyone's mind that meant it had started there and by implication it was obviously my staff's negligence that had caused it. These were views in part shared by the company, as well as the grieving relatives of the deceased, who had by now got wind of the fact that I had returned and were besieging the company offices. I made my phone calls back to London and then had to be smuggled out of a back door to avoid being lynched before I flew back home to face the press gathered outside my home.

Contemporary newspaper reports all state that the fire was first noticed in the salon and the public, always looking for someone to blame, put two and two together, made five and blamed me, just like the grieving relatives outside the Greek Line offices. This was despite the fact that the salon had actually been closed for the best part of four hours before the fire was noticed. Surely if a fire had started through my staff's negligence it would have taken hold a lot earlier.

I had lost everything. I didn't have enough insurance to cover my equipment losses and I hadn't thought to cover the risk of a catastrophe such as sinking as a result of a fire because it was such an unheard of event. I even lost the takings from the till as they too went to the bottom with the ship.

The Greek Merchant Marine authorities launched an enquiry. It lasted for two years and was based almost entirely on witness statements as all the material evidence was at the bottom of the Atlantic. During those two years, relatives of the deceased attempted to sue me left, right and centre. At one point my solicitor, a good friend of mine, wouldn't tell me how many lawsuits he had received as he was genuinely scared I'd put my head in the gas oven.

The enquiry concluded that the Lakonia should never have passed her safety inspection prior to leaving Southampton. The enquiry also argued that all of the lifeboats should have been lowered during the drill and not just five; that there were not enough responsible officers on deck to supervise the evacuation with not enough being done to evacuate passengers from their cabins. There were in fact so many safety failings that the disaster had extensive ramifications for the future of marine safety legislation and the SOLAS (Safety Of Life At Sea) regulations were amended with the enquiry findings in mind. Eight crewmembers were charged with negligence and Captain Zarbis; the ship's security officer and the first officer were all charged with gross negligence. I think Zarbis served a jail term.

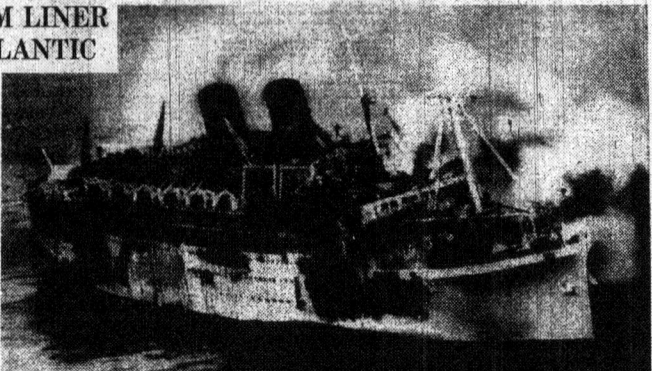

The restrained coverage of the Lakonia disaster by The Daily Telegraph on Christmas Eve 1963. You can make out the smoke billowing from the port side of the liner and a lifeboat still hanging from its davit. By kind permission of The Daily Telegraph.

After all the available evidence was considered, the enquiry concluded that the cause of the fire was most likely an electrical short circuit in the engine room. The subsequent fire was conducted up the aft stack, which passed through the barbershop. There it burst through the thin bulkhead, igniting the flammable hairdressing materials we had stored there. We had not caused the fire; I was officially exonerated.

Although the fire was never mentioned in any commercial dealings I had subsequent to the enquiry being published, the mud that had been thrown beforehand had obviously stuck with some people. Around four years after the tragedy I was on a ferry to Le Havre with a business associate. We were eating lunch and had been discussing the fire. When the waiter came to serve me he splashed the food down in front of me causing everyone to look up. He called me a bastard and hoped I'd rot in hell for killing his brother on the Lakonia. He'd heard what we were talking about, guessed who I was and obviously still harboured a grudge he could no longer contain. As I mentioned earlier, the shipping world is a small one through which gossip and rumour can travel like wildfire and reputations can be ruined as quickly as they are gained.

Chapter 19
After The Fire

I was determined that I would recover from this tragedy and that I would do it through sheer hard work, motivated by the fact that I knew I was blameless and that the truth would eventually come out. I remembered my father and the flags he'd bought on a whim and how he'd turned adversity into an advantage so I resolved that never again would I give up on anything without first giving it my all. I had been lucky in that I had already got a contract with Typaldos on a couple of their ships, the Athinai and the Akropolis, both splendid old American Grace Line ships and like sailing on time machines. While for that first couple of years after the Lakonia I was almost persona non grata in the industry, Typaldos didn't much care for reputations, deserved or otherwise. In truth, they probably suspected what had really happened on the Lakonia as they were aware of all the strokes that were pulled in the industry and knew it wasn't me to blame. So as long as I didn't set fire to their ships, I had a contract. It wasn't perfect but at least I still had work. More importantly, I was gaining a more than valuable insight into the machinations of the Greek shipping industry and this would serve me well in the coming decade.

Things came to a head with Typaldos when my staff started complaining about the conditions they were being forced to live in and the food they were having to eat. Understandably they were threatening to quit over it so I had to do something. I'd heard the owner's brother-in-law, a thoroughly unpleasant man called Kokanos, was on board so I went in search of him, eventually tracking him down to the galley where he was inspecting the food being prepared. I was aghast: he was testing the food by sticking his hand in and trying it. I just looked at him and told him straight: "You know, you not only look like a pig but you act like one. Don't bother to tell me my contract's up, I'm quitting. Goodbye." Typaldos Lines eventually went bankrupt in 1968 and I can't say I was either surprised or sympathetic.

By the time I left Typaldos my name had been cleared and I had already set off in pursuit of more work. I'd been to Italy where I had made contact with a small Italian concern by the name of Cogedar Line. They operated two ships, the Flavia and the Aurelia, on the immigrant runs to Australia from Southampton and stopping at points in between. Although they were only a tiny line, the connections I was able to make through working for them meant they were one of the most important companies I was associated with; the springboard to bigger challenges.

I developed a good friendship with the owner, a nice guy by the name of Massimo Garello. Massimo reckoned I wasn't just a hairdresser but had a good head for business with an entrepreneurial streak that was worth taking advantage of. He often used to ask my opinion and ideas on various shipping matters, especially now that I had been in the business for a few years and seen a few things.

In the summer, the Aurelia was chartered to another company to operate student trips to and from New York. Between the end of her regular runs to Australia and New Zealand and the start of the New York runs there was a ten day lay-up period during which the ship was idle and not earning anything. Massimo asked me if I had any ideas and it just so happens that I did; I suggested doing a ten-day cruise around the Med. Massimo thought about it but wondered how he could promote it. I told him I also had an idea for that, too.

At that time I had my training salon in Knightsbridge, above a chemist shop opposite where Bowater House used to be. Here I used to assess new staff and train them for the rigours of the offshore life. We had all sorts of clients coming in, from shopgirls to titled aristos presumably short of a few bob as, being a training school, we were only charging 2/6 (12.5p) a time. I had found out that the husband of one of these ladies ran a travel company and that he just happened to be the main agent for Chandris Line, one of the biggest of the Greek lines. This was potentially a very big opening for me so I went to see him and told him about the ten-day cruise. We both went over to Italy to see Cogedar and clinched the deal. In return for the business, the agent offered me £5 commission on every booking he took for the cruise but I declined, telling him that the best commission he could give me would be to arrange an introduction to Chandris Line. My foresight paid off; he arranged the meeting and Coiffeur Transocean ended up with a contract for every Chandris vessel.

That first cruise round the Med for Cogedar was quite eventful. We arrived at Algiers and as it was an overnight stopover I decided it would be good to get away from the ship for a night in a hotel. I'd been chatting to an attractive lady passenger and she asked me what I was planning on doing. I told her I was going ashore to a good restaurant then a nightclub and back to a hotel. She asked me if she could join me so I said that would be OK as long as she didn't mind sharing the room with me as I wasn't paying for two! Well, my marriage had ended by this time so I was a free agent once more!

We had a great night out and did indeed share the room. At 8am the next morning we were woken from our still deep and satisfied sleep by the telephone ringing. It was the manager asking me whether I could come down to reception. I refused, pointing out the time. He countered by telling me there were some policemen there who wanted a word with me about my identity papers. This might be a bit of a problem as I'd left my passport on the ship. We hurriedly dressed and went down. The policeman in charge explained that we'd actually entered the country illegally and asked us where our passports were because we hadn't left them at reception as we were obliged to do. We'd broken the law so it was a fair cop. We would have to go to the station but I was worried that we would miss the ship and get into even more trouble. Annoyingly, the policeman refused to accompany us back to the ship to retrieve our passports so it was beginning to look bad for us. I looked at him and thought to myself that he must be corrupt somehow so I guessed at his price.

"I must tell you," I said chancing my arm, "The whisky is very good on board."

"Is it?"

"Come on then, let's go to the ship."

When we arrived back at the Aurelia I grabbed the purser and asked him to quickly fetch a couple bottles of Scotch and to charge them to me. When he asked why, I told him to fetch our passports as well. He understood!

The following year we did a similar cruise during the lay-up but this time we went around the North Cape to Copenhagen. Because he reckoned I had all the right background and experience, Massimo asked me to be the cruise director, which meant I would also be in charge of all the entertainment as well as my own business. I set about recruiting cruise and entertainments staff and when I was done I went to Garello to ask him a favour.

"Massimo, you've asked me to do all this for you, now I want something from you in return. I'd like my parents to do this cruise and I'd like them to have the owner's suite."

"But I'm on the cruise."

"OK. Next door to you then."

"You've got it!"

-ooOoo-

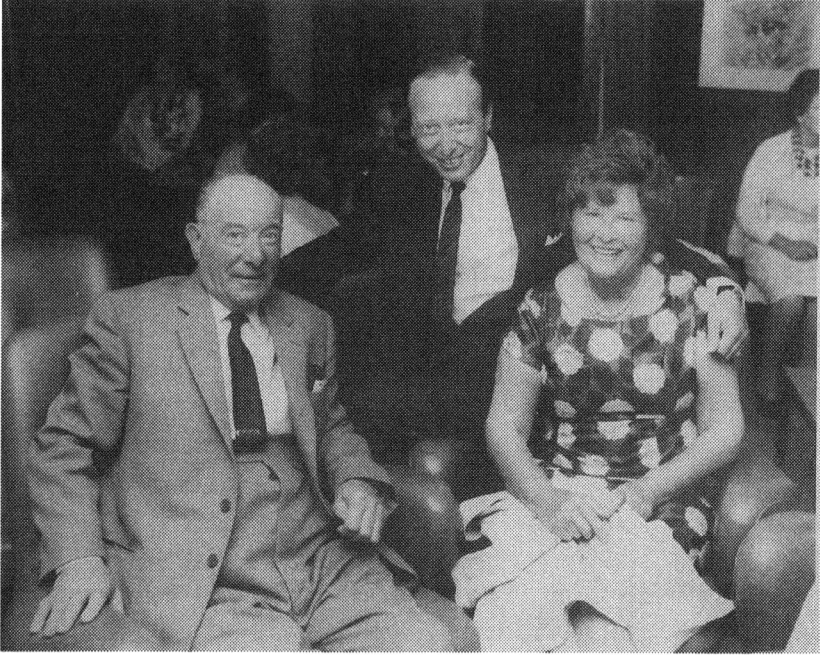

My parents on board the Aurelia

I was in a meeting one day during that cruise when my father came in asking if he could see me for a minute. When I asked him if it could wait because I was a bit busy he told me that no, it was rather important. I excused myself, wondering what on earth could be so important that he had to interrupt a meeting to tell me. I was actually a bit worried. He took me along a corridor to a staircase and pointed to a piece of carpet that had lifted.

"So what?"

"The carpet's loose, people will fall down and they'll sue you."

"They won't sue me, they'll sue the owner!"

I don't think my father quite understood my status and I'm convinced he thought I actually owned the ship.

I had a salon manager on that cruise called Garry Morris who was a bit of a character. He also suffered terribly from seasickness, usually being ill even before the ship had left port. Once I walked into the salon and there was a woman at the basin waiting to be shampooed. I couldn't see Garry anywhere so I asked her if everything was OK.

"Yes, thank you. Such a charming man, he's just gone to get some towels."

Well, I could see a pile of towels behind her so I knew where he'd gone and the ship was still in port! I offered to take over as I said I could see a few towels I could use. As I finished shampooing her Garry walked in, looking quite pale.

"Thank you, Mr Anthony, most kind of you." And he took over. Later that day I was having a drink with the captain and the purser and the same woman came in to the lounge then stopped and stared at me. Apologising to the captain she addressed me:

"I'm sorry to interrupt you, sir, but the hairdresser told me you were his apprentice" She obviously couldn't possibly understand why an apprentice would be drinking with the captain! Years later Garry went to work in America and after working as a car valet while doing the mandatory six months at school to get his licence (he obviously wasn't as lucky as I was in New York), he opened a salon in Hollywood becoming very successful. One of his clients was Lucille Ball of "I Love Lucy" fame, and a very influential Hollywood figure at the time. I visited him in LA years later and he insisted on picking me up from the airport in his Rolls Royce. I think he did OK for himself!

I was constantly writing to shipping companies and I had written to Norwegian America Line telling them I would soon be in Oslo and asking whether I could make an appointment to meet with them. They agreed. My mother asked me where I was going and when I told her that I was just off to have a meeting she told me I looked very smart with my suit and briefcase and that she was sure they would give me a contract. She was right, too as I came out of the meeting with a contract for the Oslofjord.

In those early days of the Greek companies moving into the cruise business they were often looked upon rather disdainfully by the older and more established lines. Many of their early cruise liners were old ferries and they did minimal conversion work with regard to cabin comfort and often the beds were little more than bunks with a side rail to stop you from falling out. They were nothing like the luxurious ships of today. Likewise, anyone associated with them, such as me, was treated as a Mickey Mouse operation so getting the break with NAL was a triumph. Thereafter the major companies saw me in a different light.

Chapter 20

The English Greek

I mentioned my training salon above the chemist's shop in Knightsbridge. I opened it in 1963 when I started Coiffeur Transocean and I can well remember walking up the stairs to it when I heard that JFK had been assassinated, exactly a month before the Lakonia episode. The things that came from that salon could fill a book of their own. I've often thought they'd make a good TV series but I think it would have to go out after the watershed.

One of the kids I had up there was a young lad called David Love. He was usually very good but on one particular occasion he cocked up a bit when he put the wrong colour in a South American woman's hair. She started to play merry hell so I tried to placate her by telling her that she must remember that she was in a school of hairdressing and that mistakes will inevitably happen. I asked her to come over to the basin and got David to re-colour her hair and it worked out fine. She had very long hair and as it was getting late I told David I'd finish her off so he could get himself off home to Southend.

The woman had calmed down a lot by now and was really pleased with the way her hair had turned out but that now she would also like it set. I said that as it was now quite late I would half blow-dry it, put some rollers in and then finish her off under the dryer. After I half blow-dried it the colours showed up much better and she was even more delighted. I went round and stood in front of her and started to put a roller in a long mesh of her hair. I had my hands up in the air rolling it down when she once again said she didn't know how to thank me. Then, all in one movement she slid down off the chair, unzipped my fly and before I realised what was happening, she was giving me a blow-job. Moreover, while she was showing me her appreciation in this novel way, a double-decker bus stopped outside the window and it was close enough for those sitting on top to see right in to the salon. Which they did of course and they started cheering! Because I still had my hands in the air they thought I was joining in with them! Thankfully, not all my customers were so brazen.

The training salon was always full of interesting people. A middle-eastern gentleman attached to one of the embassies used to come in every six months with his wife and children. While his wife was under the dryer he used to sit next to her, holding her hand and kissing it constantly. They were obviously a very happy and devoted couple and it was lovely to watch the attention he lavished on his beloved. I mentioned to him that I was divorced and asked him what his secret for a happy marriage was. He said it was very simple, "I see her once a year!"

Another customer was a Lady Hodge, who used to bring her daughters in with her. She was set on her youngest going to study drama at RADA but I suggested she was a natural model and that she ought to think about doing that. Vicki Hodge did indeed go on to be a very famous model but whether I had a hand in that, I don't know. I once took her as my guest to a function organised by Chandris and the other male guests' jaws dropped when I walked in with her on my arm!

A group of women used to regularly come in and they amused me because while they all sounded terribly "House and Garden" they actually had very little. The irony being of course that I, the humble East End boy doing their hair, was doing rather well, thanks. One day one of them came in wearing a fox fur stole and in her best plummy voice asked me if I had somewhere she could put her fur. "Yes, luv," came my best Cockney reply, "We've got a kennel ahtside."

One of the other girls was going through a divorce from a distant outpost of the Guinness family. She asked me if I knew a good lawyer so I suggested the one I'd used for my own divorce. Soon after that we started going out. One night she stayed at my flat in Oslo Court and before I knew it, she had moved in. Her name was Judith and she became my second wife and was the mother of my son, Alexis who was born in 1971. Sadly the marriage only survived another year after Alexis' birth. I think I probably was the marrying kind; I always tried to make a go of it but maybe I just made two unlucky choices. A couple more bad experiences with other women I became serious over meant I never tried marriage again. As a result I've enjoyed the benefits of a single life ever since.

I tried a couple of years of therapy to try and fathom the reasons why the marriages didn't work and I did in fact learn a lot about myself. As a youngster I used to watch a lot of musicals where everyone fell in love and lived happily ever after. I'm certain I held onto this ideal into adulthood, believing in romance over reality - something that isn't always the best recipe for success in a relationship. It does seem strange to dismiss several years of marriage in just a few sentences but as I've said elsewhere, I feel there's little benefit to gain in writing about it, so I won't.

-oo0oo-

I wasn't only involved with hairdressing on the ships. Not long after I started with Chandris I heard talk that the company were unhappy with the incumbent gift shop concessionaires. This was an opportunity too good to pass up and as I had become very friendly with Mimis Chandris, the owner and many of the directors I felt able to take advantage of it. I went to the man in charge, a Captain Miaoulis, and suggested he let me take over one of the smaller shops. If he liked the way I ran it then I could run the whole fleet's shops.

The first ship they gave me was the Fiesta. It was only a small ship, in fact it was an old Isle of Man ferry they'd bought and had completed a full conversion to cruise service on and this was to be her first trip, a weekend-long cruise for Greek high society. This was also just at the start of the political turmoil in Greece that would eventually lead to the coup d'état of 1967. All the stock for the gift shop and the salon had been held up at customs as a result of the divided loyalties of various departments who delighted in countermanding each other's orders to release the goods.

I met Mimis Chandris on the quayside and he asked me whether I was ready. After I explained the situation to him he told me to follow him. We went into the customs shed where he put through a call through to none other than the prime minister. When he put the put the phone down he told me to go and wait by the ship as my goods would soon be on their way. Also, when they arrived I'd better hurry and get everything set up as the first guests wouldn't be too far behind. I did as I was told and sure enough a group of motorcycle police came heading towards me, sirens wailing and lights flashing. I immediately thought it was the first of the VIPs arriving until I saw the truck behind carrying all my supplies. In a country where much of the electorate live on remote islands, shipowners are courted by the politicians and vice-versa and I suspect Mimis was able to call in a favour or two. The gift shop was a tremendous success as well. I'd stocked it with attractive, high-class goods such as expensive perfumes and Dupont lighters and these went down very well with the VIPs.

Another incident illustrated the kind of relationship I had with Chandris. They had bought an old American President Line ship, The President Hoover and renamed it the Regina. The ship was still being fitted out as we sailed up the Adriatic from Piraeus to Venice and only had a few passengers on board apart from the builders and the naval architect. The salon was still in its original location above the lounge, which I didn't think was the best place for it but the giftshop, for which I had secured the concession, was even more poorly placed on the embarkation deck. I was having a drink in the bar with the naval architect, a Mr Dobson, and I asked him whether it would be OK to swap the two locations, especially as there weren't that many passengers on board. He said it would be fine so off I went to ask permission from the captain. He agreed with me and said he'd telex Chandris for permission. There was no reply so I told him I'd go ahead anyway, certain it would be OK. The captain was a little more reticent saying he'd turn a blind eye but on my own head be it.

I checked again with Mr Dobson that it could be done and he was still certain although there was only one problem; the occupants of the cabin next to the new salon. I went and invited them to be my guests and have some drinks in the bar with the excuse that we were doing some remedial work in the room next door. I told the barman to keep plying them with drinks until they passed out! We pressed on and it was looking good until we were heading up the Grand Canal in Venice. When the captain appeared holding a telex from Chandris that read "Tell Anthony Kaye NOT to make any changes."

"Well, Captain," I said. "Goodbye! I think I've come a bit unstuck, haven't I."

When we docked in Venice I left the ship and headed off back to London expecting my contract to be terminated. Imagine the surprise therefore when I got back into the office and found a telex waiting for me there from Mimis Chandris that just read "Congratulations. You were right." He'd actually flown to Venice to have a look for himself. I thought to myself about whether one could just walk into someone else's house and knock a few walls down because in a way, that's what I felt I'd got away with. But that kind of relationship I had with Chandris back then, I still have with Mimis' sons today. It was also a big plus to me that Mimis was a huge Anglophile. He lived in England and both his sons were educated there; in fact to hear them speak you wouldn't believe they were Greek at all. Interestingly, I would later be known in the industry as the originator of the idea of taking salons and spas out of the lower deck areas and into prime locations on the liners, making them part of the overall cruise experience and where revenue could be maximised.

The Regina used to call at Haifa where there was a large duty free warehouse from where I used get lots of my stock. One time I got a fantastic deal on some Sony radios and managed to sell the whole lot on board. Needless to say, the resultant cacophony didn't go down too well with the captain! Also on the Regina I once met the president of the Dutch airline KLM's New York operations who told me he was very impressed with the way the shop was being run. This was just as 747 Jumbo Jets were being introduced and they were pondering what to do with the upper decks on their fleet. I said I thought they'd make a good shop and ended up making a presentation to their board to that effect the next time I was in New York. We were all ready to roll with it when their accountants turned round and said bums on seats would bring in more revenue. I hope they knew best!

I enjoyed the confrontations I had with the Greek owners, especially when I was able to play them at their own game. It was a fantastic grounding for me and I became known as "The English Greek" in the trade because as well as having concessions on almost the entire Greek cruise fleet, I knew them so well (although I have to admit, I only knew a few words of the language). On one occasion I was In Pireaus when nearly all the Chandris ships and some of the Kavounides craft were in port together. I wanted a staff meeting so I got all my crew off and was walking with all thirty or so of them to a restaurant for a meeting. Now, my staff was almost wholly female and as we were walking along I bumped into the chairman and MD of Chandris, both of whom I was very good friends with. "Never mind the English Greek," one of them said. "Bloody James Bond!"

While some of their methods left a lot to be desired, what I most admired about the Greek shipping operators was their ability to make something out of nothing and their endless supply of new ideas. For instance, while the big companies ran cruise ships out of Southampton that took three days to reach the warm weather (including an often miserable and seasickness inducing crossing of the Bay of Biscay), Chandris started fly cruises. You hopped on a plane at Gatwick and two or three hours later you got on a ship in Venice so you made the most of the fine weather. They were the first to do this kind of deal and by the time the big companies wised up, Chandris had a fleet operating all over the Adriatic and the Aegean.

Another Pireaus based owner bought two old ships from P & O and brought them back to Greece for conversion to cruise ships. Halfway through he ran out of money and couldn't get credit. Facing bankruptcy, he hit on the idea of advertising cheap trips to Mecca. Pilgrims had to bring their own food and it was a bit of a nightmare as he was overloading the ships and there were often ten to a cabin, all with their own paraffin stoves. Nevertheless he made his fortune. He sold the ships for scrap and retired a multi-millionaire. I came across so many of these inventive get-rich-quick schemes

My mother always had tremendous faith in me as well as marvellous insight. I didn't have enough money to stock the gift shops so I went to the bank for a loan but they refused me because I didn't have enough collateral. I'd been sure they would give me a loan on the strength of the contracts alone but I was wrong; sometimes it doesn't pay to be over confident. Now I'd committed to a contract and couldn't deliver. I was noticeably uptight about it, too because for once, I didn't have an answer. When my mother asked what was troubling me, I explained my dilemma and she offered me the use of the deeds on their house to give to the bank for collateral. I told her I couldn't possibly take them as she'd be homeless if everything went wrong. Very calmly she told me that she knew I wouldn't fail. I couldn't sleep through worrying about her house and it was one of the most trying times of my life. She was right though, it was a success and the deeds were soon returned.

Nevertheless, it took a while for Mother to cotton on to how successful the company eventually became. On Mondays she used to go to Brighton with her two sisters where they used to sit on the prom in deckchairs, chatting. One afternoon a friend of one of my aunts came along too. After a while said she was going to have to go home because her son was coming home after a year working as a manager for a company that had hair salons on ships. Mother's ears pricked up when she heard that because, to all intents and purposes, that's just what I did. The other woman said that her son worked for a very important company and that it was very big in the business. Mother asked the company name and when she heard it was Coiffeur Transocean she exclaimed, "That's my son's company!" At which point it all clicked. She couldn't wait to tell me when she got back to London.

As for getting supplies, in those days there was strict currency control but the Bank of England recognised my status as a dollar earner and gave me freedom to purchase supplies in dollars. I had an account specially for the Bank of England showing the amount of dollars earned against what I'd spent. As shipboard currency was often in dollars, this was a distinct boon to our cash flow. As I had been granted this special privilege by the Bank of England, my own Barclays branch in Knightsbridge was naturally very pleased to have me as a customer. Because of this, in 1980 I think it was, they honoured me with a luncheon at their office in Fenchurch Street in the presence of all their directors. What a turnaround and it also provided me with a delicious moment of sweet revenge.

When I first started as "Anthony Kaye trading as Coiffeur Transocean" in 1963, I'd gone to my Barclays branch manager in Piccadilly for a loan of £250. He refused and I eventually got a loan for £100 from Mike Shaw, the owner of the chemist shop below my training salon and a friend of my brother in law. I can still remember the terms after all these years - £100 at 10% repayable in 12 instalments. When I started the gift shops I knew I'd get no joy from the bank so that's when my Mother lent me the deeds of the house. Imagine my surprise then, surrounded by all these high ranking bankers when the last director walked into the room and it was the very same manager who'd refused my loan 17 years before. Oh, Fate, I love you!

Lord Somebody or Other who was sitting next to me, with impeccable timing, had just said to me, "Anthony, it's quite brilliant: you've taken a service to the Yanks that is a dollar earner for the UK without taking any materials from the UK except your talent. Well done! How did you start?" My mind flashed back to the Shirley Temple dance routine, "Now it's my turn" I thought and, pointing toward the gentleman who'd just entered the room, told him that I'd gone to him seventeen years ago for a loan and he refused me. Now, seventeen years later I'm being honoured as a unique dollar-earner, safe in the knowledge that now you'd lend me large amounts of money. What about a young person with an idea today? Do they have to hope their parents back them or do you have managers with insight nowadays," pointing again. "Unlike this gentleman?" It felt great to see him squirm, just like I had done in front of him all those years ago.

Chapter 21
Life Afloat

Despite spending so much time on ships it took me a long time to get my sea-legs. I think I finally got them through necessity more than anything else. We were crossing the Atlantic on the Regina on the way to the Bahamas for a season of Carribean cruising and it was a rough trip. The crates containing the supplies for the salon and the shop were in the forward hold, where the pitch is greatest, and I was down there with my staff busily trying to unpack them. Imagine bending down inside a crate as the bow of the ship pitches down with the swell and then rises again. You're thrown into the crate one second and the next you're ejected from it with an armful of stock and trying to keep your breakfast down. Most of the staff had to keep excusing themselves to go up on deck as they were suffering from different degrees of sea-sickness but I was determined to tough it out and stay down there as we needed everything ready by the time we reached Nassau. I was a good sailor after that trip.

To be honest, I've never really been very happy near seawater. I had developed a fear of it, and of swimming in it, after being badly stung by a big jellyfish while paddling in Westcliffe-on-Sea when I was about 4. The pain was awful and I had weals all over my legs. Ever since that day I've been scared of seawater. Many years later I was laying on a beach somewhere and my feet were just in the water. Suddenly I felt something biting me and I was terrified. I looked down and there were tiny little fish nibbling at my toes. I screamed and ran out of the water! Rather ironic to think I would eventually spend over half my life depending on the sea for my livelihood. I was a sound swimmer in a pool though and did lots of certificates when I was a kid, even getting a special one from the headmaster "for courage and determination" after cramping up while doing a longer swim than I knew I was capable of. Despite the cramp I managed to hang on to the end but I couldn't grab the railing with my bent up hands so they had to fish me out.

-oo0oo-

That season of Caribbean cruising was one of my first exposures to the excesses of some of the passengers and provided a fund of amusing memories. In the Bahamas the ship brought on a doctor from America. I've always been a great observer of people and the way some of the Americans behaved was almost beyond belief when faced with the amount of food available on board.

They would have breakfast and then have lunch in the dining room or if they didn't want to eat in the dining room they could go up on deck for a buffet. Some passengers would hurry through lunch in the dining room and then rush up on deck for the buffet before it ended. They would do the same at dinner and then find even more space to cram in some more from the midnight buffet. I didn't know if it was the sea air or whether they were just greedy.

I was sitting with the doctor one day when a gentleman who could only be described as fat walked up. He apologised for troubling us but then told the doctor: "Gee, I got such pains in my stomach. What can you give me?" The doctor gave him a disdainful look. "My friend," he said, "stop eating because you're beginning to look like a pig as well as act like one!" Chandris realised after the first cruise that they'd made a huge mistake in making all this food available because they'd eat everything in sight. They never stopped.

We also had some of the early Slendertone machines on board. These are faradic muscle exercising machines that stimulate muscles using minute electric charges delivered through electrodes attached to the skin with sticky pads. They're quite common now and Slendertone is a well-known company but they were still something of a novelty 40 years ago. As I was also trying to sell the machines I decided to take the portable model out on deck and hired an attractive girl to demonstrate it while wearing a bikini. This strategy worked and she did indeed boost sales. She was ever such a well spoken girl though and when I came on board to ask how it was going she told me in her cut-glass English accent that it was getting quite interesting. "But there's one thing that's been bothering me."

"What's that then?" I asked, intrigued.

"These damn crew members! Every time they walk past they do this. What on earth does it mean?" She then proceeded to demonstrate the time honoured bent arm, clenched fist and clutched bicep signal commonly used by young gentleman signifying their approval of a young lady's charms.

"Well my dear," I said, "It means they want to fuck you!"

"Oh. Does it? How interesting." I walked off, leaving her to it. I came back a bit later only to watch her call out, "I say!" to two crewmen as they walked past. When they turned round she gave them the salute in return. It was hilarious watching them hare off. The girl eventually married into the gentry and I think became a countess!

One night on board the Regina I was asleep in my cabin when suddenly I heard shouting and footsteps running along the corridor. Fearing another Lakonia I leapt out of bed and opened the door only to find nobody there. I thought I must have been dreaming so I went back to bed. Once again it happened and once more I jumped out of bed and found nothing. Next morning I had to go to the purser's office and he asked me whether I'd been woken by the noise during the night. I told him I had and asked him what had happened. It transpired that in a cabin near me was an elderly man with a much younger girlfriend. Unfortunately he wasn't very well endowed so in an effort to impress his young love he was wearing a ring around his shaft in order to keep his swollen member in a rather more engorged state than it was designed to be. He'd been a little over-zealous in his choice of ring and gone too small and alarmingly the ring had actually cut off the blood supply to his penis, keeping it swollen. This meant he couldn't get it off. The first set of footsteps running past my cabin belonged to the ship's doctor; he couldn't shift it. The second set was none other than the ship's plumber, presumably with a set of tin-snips. Apparently the amorous old gent was so embarrassed he left the ship the next morning.

That Caribbean cruise on board the Regina allowed me to indulge another one of my passions. We'd stopped in Port of Spain, Trinidad and it just so happened that there was a cricket test between West Indies and MCC on. No question about it, I had to get in even though I knew it would be packed solid, as they love their cricket in Trinidad. The ground is the Queen's Park Oval so, just like back in London, I hailed a taxi and asked the driver to take me to the Oval.

"You got a ticket, Boss?" He asked. "You won't get in otherwise as they'll close the gates." I told him that no, I didn't have a ticket but that it didn't matter. As we neared the ground he told me again that I would be wasting my time. I asked him if he was a betting man and he said he was partial to a little flutter now and again. Then I asked him to recommend a good restaurant. Now puzzled, he replied that there was a great Chinese restaurant nearby. So I told him that if I didn't get into the Oval, I'd buy him dinner at the Chinese restaurant.

"Man, you got a bet!"

I asked him to take me round to the members' entrance. When we arrived, there were four mounted policeman outside and a large padlock on the gate. I told my new friend the driver to wait and watch as I walked up to the policemen. "Gentlemen," I said in my best posh. "You're doing a fine job there. I'm very proud to see you've got this under control. Now, I've just arrived from London. Would you be kind enough to let me in?"

"Are you a member, sir?"

"Of course. Not only am I a member but I've been very concerned by the security arrangements and I'm very pleased you've got it right." And with that, they called for the doorman. I shouted back to the taxi driver: "See you in the restaurant!" And I watched him banging his head on the steering wheel in disbelief. My only problem now was that I was in but I had nowhere to sit. They were hanging out of the trees it was so packed. Every now and then someone would shake a tree and people would change places. I wasn't going up a tree so I tried something else. "Come on guys and girls, make way for a limey!" And everyone shuffled about and made a space for me between a man on one side and a lady on the other. West Indies were batting and as I sat down someone hit a boundary and the crowd all rose and cheered as only West Indian crowds do. Unfortunately this meant I had two elbows dig into my ribs. Never mind, I was in and the atmosphere was great. I had a great time and it's probably the funniest day I've spent at a cricket match. Not only did I have the two characters flanking me but there were the cigarette sellers walking up and down, themselves genuine characters. They sold du Maurier cigarettes, which I hadn't seen in England for years. "Get your du Mauriers here!" they would cry.

"Get out the way, we can't see!"

"Buy my cigarettes and I'll move."

When I came out after a terrific day's cricket the taxi driver was waiting for me. "Does this mean I got to buy you dinner?" I told him that I valued and appreciated his honesty so much that I would buy us both dinner. "Man," he said. "I'm gonna tell my children this because I've never seen this before!"

I do seem to have this ability to sweet-talk myself into or out of situations quite easily. Back with Royal Caribbean for example their directors were boasting that they had set up tight security. I bet them $20 I could get on board without using any ID because I didn't think their security was tight at all. They didn't believe me so I told them to watch.

I walked up the gangway and immediately two security guards challenged me. Unfazed, I spoke to them confidently, politely and with authority.

"Good morning, gentlemen" I enquired, "Is everything OK here?"

"Why sir?"

"Well I want to know if you've had any problems since you've been here today. Have you had anyone who's been difficult?"

"No, sir."

"Are you absolutely sure?"

"Yes, sir."

I carried on with this officious tone for a short while until I said, "Now, carry on." And walked straight past them carrying my briefcase. There wasn't a challenge in sight or earshot. The directors were waiting for me in the purser's lobby and they said that what they'd seen was ridiculous. I told them it wasn't, it was just psychology at work. If somebody had a determined, positive and aggressively authoritative demeanour they probably won't be challenged. They changed their security arrangements on the strength of my demonstration.

I don't know whether it was the legacy of learning hypnosis that made me able to apply a bit of psychology and make myself convincing or just an acute sense of knowing what is the right thing to do in a given situation. Certainly when we got the concession on the Costa Line flagship, the Eugenio C, I needed all my powers of persuasion to prevent a "situation" from developing.

We arrived at Genoa to take the concession over only to find the whole crew out on strike. Moreover, the owners, the Costa family, told me they were on strike because of me. It turned out that the ship's barber was the union shop steward and because the salon staff were all being replaced with English staff, they all went on strike. I asked Costa if they wanted me to speak to the barber because I knew what his game was.

We knew he'd been fiddling and he knew that the moment we went on board revenue would go up because the fiddling would stop and he'd be found out. I asked him whether the strike was called because of an English crew coming on board or whether it was because he was coming off. Then I told him that if he wanted to stay on board I would recommend that he run the barbershop and not only that, he could keep all the takings. He thought it sounded good but he wondered what I meant by keeping all. I levelled with him and said I knew he was on the take but that I was prepared to let him have all of it. He called off the strike immediately. He'd only be making money off his crew mates as male passengers rarely used the barbershop so salon takings would easily cover any shortfall. Situation averted!

-ooOoo-

By 1968 I had got several more gift shop concessions but it now started to get a little bit too much for me. Running the shipboard salons was work enough but I also had my training salon and the office to run back in London and on top of that I was chief cook and bottle-washer for the shops. I was responsible for finding qualified staff to run them and then I was the buyer, constantly visiting suppliers in different countries and then working out the retail prices. I desperately needed help. I mentioned it to my solicitor who said he had an American client called Ron Franklin who was an experienced retailer in the department store business and who he thought he would make an ideal partner to run the Transocean gift shops. Ron and I met and we made a deal for him to take a 50% share in the shops and to run them. I decided though that I wanted to keep the salons under my personal control.

Chapter 22
Car Trouble

My new partner, Ron, and I flew out to Athens to do a stock inventory. Greece was now being governed by the military junta of Colonel Papadopoulos and the government had stopped foreign currency from leaving the country. There was a lot of money on the ships because we had told the staff not to bank money in Greece as we would have a devil of a time getting it back out. Instead, we transferred the money to the Fantasia, on which we were due to sail to Venice. It turned out to be an eventful trip in more ways than one. Not least because Ron and I were accompanied by one of my hairdressers, a very beautiful Norwegian girl, who was transferring to another ship.

After we set sail I had a message from the captain inviting us to his quarters for cocktails. Now, I knew the captain very well and I knew what he was after; he'd seen my girl and was interested in her. I also thought there was a chance for a bit of fun at his expense so I told her what to expect and along we went to be entertained. Needless to say, he wasn't successful in his amorous quest that night. It was a three-day voyage though so he didn't give up trying and on the Captain's Dinner night we were invited along to his quarters again.

This time he thought that I was the reason for his lack of success and kept plying me with drinks in order to get me drunk and incapable. What he didn't know was that when he wasn't looking, in time-honoured sitcom style, I was tipping the drinks into his plant pots. I then went into his bedroom and reappeared wearing his tunic saying that I should go to his table in place of him so that he could have dinner with the girl in his quarters. He thought it was a great idea, so I dressed up in the full uniform and joined the other passengers at the captain's table.

All the other passengers were English and they were very surprised when the captain didn't turn up. When they asked where he was I told them he had been taken ill and had had to leave the ship. They wanted to know how an English captain could command a Greek vessel. I told them I would show them how during the dessert course. The crew knew what was happening and were having difficulty containing their laughter when they brought out the flaming baked alaskas. I uttered my few words of Greek and they all stood to attention and said in unison and in English, "We hope you have enjoyed your cruise" which impressed the passengers no end. Needless to say, the real captain still had no success with the hairdresser.

I didn't let up when we arrived in Venice, either. I sent a cable to the captain that appeared to come from the Norwegian girl. "She" apologised for not being able to spend more time with him but that there would be a girlfriend of hers sailing on the next cruise, in cabin 409, and that she had been told to look out for him. It was a pack of lies of course and when the captain went to check cabin 409, he found it was occupied by a married couple.

When we arrived at Venice, Ron and I hired a car so we could drive across the country to Genoa in order to complete the inventory on the ships there. The Norwegian girl was still with us as the ship to which she was transferring was also berthed there. We stopped just outside Milan for petrol and a coffee around 9am then headed back out onto the autostrada.

I was driving fast to make up time and went to overtake the car in front when it suddenly pulled out on me. Going too fast to hit the brakes, I swung the wheel to avoid hitting him but I lost control and we ended up on the wrong side of the road. There was a car coming straight at me so I tried to steer back to our side of the road. I didn't make it in time and the oncoming car hit my driver's door. I wasn't wearing a seatbelt and as the car spun round I was thrown headfirst through the windscreen fracturing my skull when my head hit the road. Amazingly, even though the car had turned over three times, Ron and the girl escaped serious injury. Afterwards I found out that she knew we were carrying the money and that she would not leave the scene of the accident until the firemen had jemmied open the boot allowing her to recover the money for me.

I was in hospital in Italy for two weeks. When I regained consciousness after three days I didn't know where I was and I thought I was dreaming. There were all these blurred ladies in white around me who appeared to be genuflecting before me. I thought that I was in heaven surrounded by angels rather than an Italian hospital being attended to by nurses. Nobody spoke English and I was trying to find out where I was. Ron was outside and having heard that I was awake, entered the room and told me what had happened to me.

I had an unbearable headache and when the doctor came in I tried to tell him about it in the few words of Italian I knew. He went out and came back with two Aspirin. Talk about incompetence. After eight days they decided to x-ray me and later, when the doctor came back into my room with the plates, he told me in reasonable English that the reason I had a pain in my head was that my skull was fractured from front to back. It had taken them over a week to work this out. By now I was also becoming paralysed down my right side so I got Ron to phone my London manager to ask my own doctor there to find a neurologist who could see me.

He found one in Milan and he came to visit me. He took one look at the X-rays and said that I should get out of that hospital quickly because they didn't know how to deal with my condition. My manager flew over from London and he booked a flight back for me with BEA. The only problem was, they didn't have room for a stretcher on their Milan flight, only from Turin 100 miles away and we'd have to get there by road. The ambulance he hired for the transfer was a rickety little thing, barely able to take the stretcher and my manager. I was amazed that I arrived at Turin airport at all because all it seemed to do for the duration of the journey was bounce around wildly.

BEA had taken out the seats at the front of the plane for the stretcher and once we were airborne I thought I could smell eggs and bacon. The food in the hospital had been of the usual inedible standard despite it being in a country with a renowned cuisine, so I asked the hostess whether the gorgeous aromas I could smell were for real. I wasn't imagining it and she asked me if I wanted breakfast. I said yes but I had to ask her to feed me as the whole of my right side, including my face, was completely useless. She was marvellous; she got down on her knees and fed me and then got straws for me to drink tea through. I just wish I could remember her name.

We were met by an ambulance at Heathrow that took me to the Hospital for Nervous Diseases at Maida Vale. There the consultant examined me and, after taking many readings, told me that he was amazed I was still alive. Not only had I survived the crash but also the lack of proper treatment in the hospital, the appalling ride in the ambulance and then the flight in a pressurised aircraft. He said the prognosis was good though and that I would recover all my faculties given time. I had health insurance and asked if I could have a private room but he said there were only four and they were all in use. He could transfer me to the London Clinic but I wouldn't get the same 24 hour neurological supervision there so I stayed in the public ward. It was a nightmare with people screaming and punching the nurses while being treated so I spent most of my time devising ways of getting out.

I'd never liked hospitals, ever since I was a child and my mother took me to have my tonsils out at a hospital in Fitzroy Square where I was strapped down to the operating table with thick leather belts. When I came round after blowing into this balloon affair that had made me go to sleep, I had a terrible sore throat and all I wanted to do was vomit. Yet every time I did, a vicious sister kept appearing who slapped my face telling me not to. I also still have a scar on my thigh from a hypodermic needle used when I had scarlet fever. The thing looked as though it was more suited to a horse than a child. There seemed to be no compassion towards children in hospitals in those days.

After a month or so of this a doctor came round to do some comparative reasoning tests i.e. they would say a word and the patient answers with a word suggested by the prompt such as black:white, dog:cat etc. When he got to me, one of the prompts was "guitar" to which I replied "sex". He was curious so I told him to think of its beautiful rounded shoulders going down to a narrow waist and ending in a gorgeous curvaceous bottom; what could possibly be more sexual? He told me he thought I was now ready to go home. My work involved huge amounts of travelling and I was effectively out of action for around nine months all told before the paralysis had fully receded.

Home at the time was Oslo Court in St John's Wood. To continue with the car theme for a while, my ex-wife's brother was living with me at the time while he was studying and it was from him that I bought the number plate that still adorns my current car. It's a plate that has intrigued many over the years because it contains the number 666, the biblical number of the beast from the Book of Revelations. People have often asked me what it's like to have it or does it worry me and I can honestly say it's never bothered me. A few odd things have happened while I've been driving but certainly nothing apocalyptic. It's definitely emotive for some though: I had it on an Alfa Spyder that I drove around Europe in and when I got to the Italian border the guard wouldn't get out of his little booth. Instead he just pointed and shouted "Sei, sei, sei – speziale!" raised the barrier and shooed me on my way.

I had the plate on a terrific Volvo P1800, the car made famous by Roger Moore as Simon Templar in "The Saint", which was a hugely popular television series at that time. Driving down to Millwall Docks one summer, I got caught in a traffic jam by a block of flats. There were some kids playing nearby and of course, I got the treatment. "Cor! Look it's The Saint's car!" I can still see him now: the kid who ran across to me wore thick bottle-bottom glasses. He stuck his head in through the open window and immediately yelled back to his mates, "Yeah, it's The Saint's car alright but it ain't the bleedin' Saint drivin' it." Of course it wasn't – my one was red!

Another time I was hit up the rear by a brand new Hillman at a junction in Queensway, West London. I was stationary at the time and the whole of front the Hillman was smashed in while my car had barely suffered a scratch. I got out and asked what on earth the driver thought he was doing. He apologised and said that it wasn't really his fault. "It was hers!" he said, pointing at a girl walking along in a miniskirt and boots. This was the start of "Swinging London" and Mary Quant's new mini-skirt was driving the capital's men crazy. "I'll tell you what's worse though" he went on, "I'm a car dealer and I'm meant to be delivering this."

When I had my training salon in Knightsbridge I used to park in one of the side streets nearby (this was before meters became commonplace). One morning I parked there as usual but some scaffolding had been erected over my spot. When I returned later there was a dent in the bonnet and a note on the windscreen with a contact number for a heating engineer! When I called him later he was terribly apologetic saying, "One of my blokes was up the scaffolding when this bird in a mini skirt and boots walked past and he dropped his bloody sledgehammer right on top of your car." I'm certain the mini skirt was directly responsible for far too many stupid accidents caused by gawping men.

I was driving along the Bayswater Road one day, again in the Volvo, and in those days it was often full of 'working women', so much so that at certain times of the day (or night) it could be like a parade down there. Ahead of me today though was a bus stop and standing in the queue was a girl who used to work for me. I stopped the car and asked her if she'd like a lift. Of course she recognised me and jumped straight in. No sooner had I started to pull away then there was a whack on the back of the car. I stopped and turned round to see a policeman standing there. The noise was the sound of his helmet, which he'd thrown at the car. He came over and said that he'd told me to stop. When I asked why, he said because I'd picked up a prostitute. "Be careful what you say, officer." I said. "This lady was waiting for a bus and she also used to work for me. And what's more, I can prove it. Now I'm going to look at the damage to my car."

Chapter 23
The Mob and a Little Competition

Towards the end of the 1960s Norwegian America Line and other transatlantic operators began to realise that the scheduled Atlantic crossings were under fierce competition from faster and more affordable air travel. The two great Cunard Queens were now out of commission - the Queen Mary in Long Beach and the Queen Elizabeth at the bottom of Hong Kong Harbour (although she'd already been converted to a floating university) - so if shipping lines were to survive, they were going to have to seek out new opportunities.

There was a huge and largely untapped market for cruising the Caribbean from east coast USA and the vastly underused port of Miami was seen as a promising centre of operations. Royal Caribbean Cruises had been formed by two Norwegian freighter operators who set out to exploit this new US market. I had heard of their ambitions to operate their newbuilding ship, the Song of Norway, out of Miami and I was interested in working with them so I flew out there to meet them. Even though their ideas were all still only drawings on a board, I thought they had something and we negotiated a contract. Some in the industry thought I was on a hiding to nothing as they saw Miami as little more than a one-horse-town because only a couple of ships ever stopped there. Now of course, it's one of the biggest and busiest ports in the world. It was a fortuitous alliance as Coiffeur Transocean also grew with Royal Caribbean as I was seen as being almost part and parcel of their operation.

Ron and I had a few differences regarding the gift shops business and I ended up giving him first refusal on my half of it, which he accepted. Before we parted company though he said I ought to meet a New York based businessman called Ellie Shallit, who was very well connected in the shipping world, because he had some contacts who may be able to put some business my way.

I arranged to meet him in New York and it was like meeting my grandfather. He was concerned whether I had eaten enough even though I'd just flown in from London and after more food he asked me if I wanted to expand into some more land based salons. I was always happy to expand, I told him, so he said he would put me in touch with some people in Miami who were interested in my business and that he would set up the meeting. I said I'd be staying at the Holiday Inn on Collins Avenue.

I had only been in the hotel a couple of hours when the phone rang. A man introduced himself and asked whether we could meet that same day. If so, he would pick me up in the lobby in half an hour. At the appointed time I went down and was gobsmacked to be greeted by the sight of the first stretch limo I'd ever seen. This was 1971 so they were hardly a commonplace sight. We drove off to the most fashionable district of Miami Beach and stopped outside one of the biggest houses. We didn't go into the house, instead we walked to the bottom of the grounds, which backed onto a waterway, and straight onto a houseboat. It was like walking on to a James Bond film set. There was a spiral staircase down which a man came running dressed in tennis kit, apologising that he couldn't see me because he'd forgotten he had a doubles match to play in. His manager had the authority to discuss everything with me and it would be just like speaking to him. After his boss had gone the manager asked me how much I thought "The Boss" was worth. I told him I hadn't a clue because I'd only seen him for a minute and then dressed up for a tennis match. He told me that he started as a kid selling papers for a dime and that now his private wealth was $50 million, a vast fortune in 1971.

He then asked me who were the biggest hair salon operators in the US and I told him: Glemby and Seligman and Latz, who each had around 3000 units mainly in department stores and shopping malls.

Then he hit me with the bombshell; they were the Jewish Mafia and they had a lot of money to invest. I hadn't a clue about money laundering back then but I was about to be introduced to the finer principles of it. He asked if I could open 500 salons a year. I replied that it was impossible and proffered a weak joke about what would happen if I only managed 499. Would I end up in a cement coffin at the bottom of the harbour? He told me that it wasn't like that at all any more, it was a bit more refined. This kind of thing was out of my league. Dodger Mullins, my father's old oppo, was the limit of my criminal connections and I certainly didn't want any trouble. I politely told him I would get back to them and left for the airport.

While waiting for my plane back to London I was looking for a book to read and I found one on the story of Israel's fight for independence. I began to read it and there was the name Ellie Shallit. The gentle and avuncular man I'd met in New York who was now a respected figure in the shipping world, had at one time allegedly been connected with the illegal shipment of arms to Israel. With the collusion of the dockers' unions it had been sent to the Middle East labelled as farm equipment. The FBI got onto him and he'd fled to Mexico to escape arrest. A fascinating story but also a scary one. There was no suggestion that any violence would be involved by these new contacts of Mr Shallit's, or for that matter that he even had any knowledge of their activities, but I often wonder what would have happened to me had I chosen to work with them.

I almost invariably managed to cultivate good business relationships with the shipowners and because I had managed to get involved at the greasy end of operations, so to speak, as well as the commercial side, they respected my knowledge and experience of the whole business. To them, I wasn't just a salon owner and they would often ask my advice or pump me for ideas.

Ted Arison was somebody I'd known for a few years. He had started out with a booking company and then moved into the cruise operator business himself in 1971, basing himself in Miami. He had bought the Empress of Canada from Canadian Pacific Line as his first ship and it was being converted at Tilbury. He knew that I had an operation on the Empress of Canada's sister ship, built as the Empress of Britain but then run by Greek Line as the Queen Anna Maria, so he asked me over to Tilbury to view his purchase, which had been renamed the Mardi Gras. He offered me a contract for the hairdressing concession and a few months later I went over to Miami to sign it.

Feeling like we were acting out a scene from "On the Waterfront" or similar, we were sitting in Ted's car in the largely freight Miami docks and I was reading the contract. It appeared to tie me exclusively to Ted's company, Carnival, which at that time only had the one ship. I told him there and then that I was sure he would have more ships in the future but that I had many other contracts to honour and couldn't tie myself to such a tiny operation. Ted took one look at the contract and tore it up before flinging it out of the window into the harbour, saying it was the wrong one, it was for the catering concession. Little did I know that my off-the-cuff prophesy would come true for Ted. Not only did he buy the Queen Anna Maria as his second vessel and rename it the Carnivale when Greek Line went to the wall in 1975, Carnival Cruise Lines, his company, would eventually become the largest cruise company in the world. They would, among others, own both Cunard and P & O and Ted would become the 10th wealthiest man in America and purportedly, the world's wealthiest Jew!

He didn't make much out of me though because I found it very difficult to work alongside some of the staff he'd brought in and the business methods they employed so I bought myself out of the contract. It was later taken up by my main competitors. Ted struck a hard bargain in business but out of the boardroom was a delightful man. Often I would arrive at his office and instead of being sent in by his secretary, Ted always came out and greeted me. He and I remained firm friends until his death in Israel, where he'd moved to in 1990, in 1998.

-oo0oo-

I mentioned my main competitor. All through my time afloat this was a company called Steiner and it is fairly safe to say our relationship was based on a more than healthy rivalry. There was very little love lost between us but I was always at a loss to explain their apparent animosity towards me. As a company they were far older than Coiffeur Transocean, having had land based salons for many years; they were also well established in the shipping world before I came along. I however, had forged good relationships with the lines in double quick time so maybe they were quite right to see me as a fast growing threat.

I got wind of their opinion of me around the beginning of the 1970s when Cunard were building some new ships, among them the Cunard Ambassador and the Adventurer. As I was signing the contract Cunard had offered me, their director turned to me and said, "By the way, I had a phone call from Steiner's a little while ago and they were furious. They asked how we could give a contract to a tuppenny-ha'penny company. What do think of that?" I told him that if I were them I would think very carefully about what we'd just said. If Coiffeur Transocean were a tuppenny-ha'penny company and they got the contract, then we must be worth even less."

"Rather clever!" was his reply.

Whenever we got new contracts in a fleet where Steiner had a foothold I was told we had to adhere to their prices as they were the bigger company but often it wasn't long before it was the other way round.

I felt they had a fear of me. I was always coming up with new ideas ahead of them and once they'd caught up with me I was away on a different project but I'm certain that their dislike of me stemmed from a meeting one of their chief executives had with Royal Caribbean Cruise Line. The Royal Caribbean Vice President of Operations, who was a good friend of mine, on asking why, if Steiners were so successful they only had a concession on one Princess Cruises ship against my two, received a reply that shocked him. He was told that it was because I had bribed their executives. He asked the Steiner rep whether he was also insinuating that I was bribing him because I had secured the whole Royal Caribbean fleet and he promptly threw him out of the office.

Naturally I heard about this exchange so I decided I would bring this up with the same executive at a meeting that had already been arranged at their Mayfair salon. I was already fired up because the meeting was actually on a completely different matter: we had arranged a route swap and as a goodwill gesture I had to purchase some of Steiner's equipment that was on the vessel we were taking over. When I walked into the office I was met with, "Ah, finally we two gladiators meet!"

"My dear friend," I countered, "gladiators fight honourably."

"What do you mean?"

"Exactly what you heard; gladiators fight with honour. You, my dear friend, have been underhand by accusing me of bribing executives and I want a written apology otherwise I'll see you in court."

Two days later I received a letter of apology but it was never the same after that episode and there always seemed to be a constant level of acrimony on their part. It didn't stop them snapping up the routes I'd given up as being either unprofitable or difficult to run, as happened when I gave up the Costa Line ships because of the chopping and changing that went on with their itineraries. My finance director said that if we gave them up, Steiners will take them but as far as I was concerned, that was a perfectly sound business decision as they would have their hands full with them, allowing us to expand. Being one jump ahead was what it was all about and all's fair in business. And of course, I couldn't really blame them for being wary of me, I was doing very well!

Chapter 24
Family

The company continued to grow throughout the 1970s. I also had several land-based salons in hotels in the UK and around the world. We had a salon in the Fred Olsen Hotel in Lanzarote, the Cunard Hotel in St Lucia and the Hilton Hotels in Kensington, West London; Stratford upon Avon and Basle in Switzerland. The last one was quite ridiculous as the prices were just unbelievable. I told the architect, who was also the designer, that he was putting the chairs too close together and that there would be no room for the stylists to work back-to-back. He said that with rent at the price per square metre it was in Basle, it would be cheaper for the stylists to all turn together!

The enjoyment of those early 70s years as the company went from strength to strength was tempered by the loss of my mother in August 1972. She had had a heart attack and was in hospital when I had to go to Copenhagen for the naming ceremony of the Royal Viking Star, the first of the three Royal Viking ships. Her doctor had told me she was fine and, as I was only going to be away for a day, it would be OK to leave her. She did indeed look great, even the nurses agreed how well she looked. She said she felt fine too and that I should go so I felt happier about leaving her. As I walked up the gangway to the ship the Chief Purser met me with a cablegram and my heart sank. My feelings as I read the news that she had passed away instantly from an even bigger heart attack than the first one were the worst I'd ever known; I felt that half of me had died because we were so close. It was made even worse by knowing she'd looked so well when I'd left for Denmark.

My father died ten years later and it's a measure of the lack of respect I'd built up for him over the years that I can't even remember the date. Much of the remainder of any feeling I had for him had gone during Mother's illness and his lack of care was verging on the cruel. Her illness caused her to have periods of dementia and also incontinence. A nurse was living in to take care of her and she told me she was having trouble keeping mother clean because of the lack of hot water. I said there should be plenty of water but she once again denied it, saying that the boiler had broken and Father wouldn't let anyone in to fix it in case he got ripped off. Instead he'd told her to use the old geyser boiler in the bathroom.

I was furious with him. I demanded to know what kind of man he was, that he could deny his wife, my mother, the hot water she needed all day. I phoned the gas board and told them it was an emergency and that I'd pay extra to get them to come out. My father said he wouldn't pay any extra; I told him I would pay but that he ought to think about what he'd done as one day he might need hot water and I might not want to pay for it. His attitude changed completely when the nurse quit and the agency sent a new one. She was very pretty and all of a sudden he became the epitome of a loving, caring husband just to impress her.

When Mother died he sent me the most vitriolic letter imaginable. He accused me of killing her with a television set. He hated TV and moreover, he hated Mother watching it, even though it was the only bit of pleasure she had left. She only had a little black and white set so I took out a contract with Radio Rentals for a 21″ colour set for her, which was a big screen in those days. She was thrilled and it made me happy to see the pleasure it was giving her. One day the set caught fire. Father pulled the plug on it and it stopped. Radio Rentals took it away and replaced it but a few days later Mother had her first attack. She'd either been forgetting to take her blood pressure tablets or deliberately not taking them. Either way, Father wasn't interested because as far as he was concerned, it was the telly causing it. He'd finally managed to kill off any last vestiges of respect I had left for him.

-oo0oo-

My late brother Bernard was an inveterate gambler and it caused much friction between us over the years. I have to say though that I never let it dissolve into bitterness and I tried to carry on helping him until the day he died of lung cancer several years ago. I'd seen what carrying resentment around for years had done to my father and I was determined I would not be like him. Sometimes I would lend Bernard money to help him out and I'd never see it again. He'd even cross the road out of embarrassment to avoid having to talk to me if he knew he owed me money.

He lost everything and had to move into my parents' house with his family. I gave my sister-in-law a job with my company and suggested Bernard take up mini-cabbing. He did and appeared to be doing well, even got himself a new home. One day he came to me asking for a loan to get a new car as his old one was falling to bits. I said that as long as it was keeping him in business, he could have the money.

A couple of days later I needed to meet a ship at Tilbury early in the morning as there was a lot of money on board owed to me and the ship was about to change hands. Alexis needed to get to nursery school in Roehampton for nine a.m. so I phoned and asked Bernard if he would mind taking him in for me but he refused saying he had to meet an important client at Heathrow at nine. I suggested he could drop Alexis off on the way a bit earlier and leave him with the teachers because he could still get there on time if he did but still he refused. "Fuck you!" I told him and hung up.

He later came round and apologised but I closed the door in his face, telling him this was the first time I'd ever asked him for help after all the help I'd given him and he'd refused. He was no longer a brother I said, but a stranger. When I went into work the next day my sister-in-law stormed into my office and had a go at me for wanting a lift for Alexis when Bernard was meeting his most important client. I've said often that I don't like talking about money but this time I let fly. I told her that she was looking at his most important client after all the help I'd given him over the years. He wouldn't even have had any clients had it not been for me buying his car for him, which was worth more than his Heathrow client would have paid him in 5 years. With that she threw her keys down and walked out. I forgave him though and as I said, I never stopped trying to help him but it was sad it involved arguments along the way.

Chapter 25
USA Again

My salons often featured in magazine articles and one I particularly remember was one by Gladys Nicol in "The Lady" in September 1973. She had travelled on the inaugural voyage of the Royal Viking Sky earlier in the year and was very impressed with the salon and the skill of the staff. Privately she told me that she was also impressed with my man management skills and that the only other person she'd met with similar ones was Harold Wilson, at that time Leader of the Opposition but until three years previously, the British Prime Minister. This wasn't surprising as we had a very good training programme and many staff worked their way through to executive positions with the company. This incentive was open to everyone in the company and it really helped to motivate the staff. I liked to promote from within as we could capitalise on the experience the staff member had accumulated as he or she climbed through the ranks.

It wasn't always smooth running though. My first foray into the American market was almost a disaster. Around 1980 American Hawaii Cruises started up, using the old American Export Lines vessel the Independence. When I went to see them about getting a contract I realised that I wouldn't get one because I wasn't an American company, so I formed one just for the one ship.

I had to have American staff, because the ship was sailing exclusively between American ports, and for some reason this just didn't work. I enlisted female masseuses from California to work in the fitness suite but they proved to lack the same kind of dedication their British counterparts did. As I often did, I went out to visit the ship to see how my new staff members were getting on. The chief officer had been conducting a lifeboat drill and he came up to me telling me that he couldn't stand it anymore as my staff were driving him crazy. He was trying to conduct a sensible drill, an important requirement on any ship, yet one my girls would arrive wearing sandals and a silly little skirt, then she would start larking around getting everyone to dance. The poor chief apparently became so paranoid that in the end he left the ship on a stretcher.

It wasn't only high jinks either. At the end of every cruise, customs used to come on board with sniffer dogs. There were drugs everywhere; absolutely anywhere they could be hidden they were found. This wasn't just my staff though, it was rife throughout the ship. I decided there and then that although having to have an American company was unavoidable, it was better to transfer contracts from the British company to the American one. I did have staff from other countries but the majority was British.

In time, the Miami arm of the operation would outgrow the London end as the cruise world began to centre itself in Florida. Over the next 15 years I would build alongside the cruise lines until I had over 500 staff on some 60 ships with another 20 or so in the Miami office and half a dozen manning the London HQ. It was an exciting time for everyone. I even had a salon on the Delta Queen, a Mississippi riverboat!

Ships created their own set of problems, it wasn't like running a land based salon at all. For example on one occasion a Norwegian America Line ship was halfway round a world cruise, Singapore or somewhere, and we got a call from the manager of the salon saying that the barber was ill and would have to come off – could we send out a replacement? I had one guy who was very good and who I was priming to become a manager so I asked him to go and fill in until the end of the cruise. I got a call from him almost the minute he arrived: "What gives with this guy who's left the ship ill? I'm a bit worried as there's long line of crewmen outside the barbershop waiting for me to come in." Apparently he'd been the backbone of the gay community on board and had caught something from one of his liaisons.

An incident involving one my beauticians on board a Royal Caribbean ship in the late 70s early 80s was like a story from Miami Vice. She had a South American boyfriend, Venezuelan I think, and he had been on holiday in Jamaica. When the ship stopped there he came on board to see her and asked her if she could keep two large boxed speakers he'd bought in her cabin until the ship arrived in Miami where he would collect them. Without thinking, she agreed. A while later the staff captain was doing his rounds, saw these two huge boxes and asked the girl what they were. She told him but the staff captain replied that it was illegal and that technically they were freight and as such they needed to be entered onto the ship's manifest so they could clear customs. He let her off but said the speakers would have to be moved to the store-room.

He went to lift up one of the boxes but it weighed a ton so he went and got two crewmen to help him. He was a bit suspicious by now as although speakers can be a bit heavy, they shouldn't be *this* heavy. He opened one of the boxes and was alarmed to see it was full of cocaine, millions of dollars worth of it. Realising the girl was almost certainly innocent he went to the captain for advice. The captain said that if they declared it right away the vessel would have to be impounded until an investigation was carried out and that this would cost the company heavily. He radioed through to Miami. The skipper wanted to dump the coke overboard but keep the boxes. That way at least they wouldn't get caught by customs at the next stopover but they could inform the Miami police in time for their arrival there. HQ agreed and when the ship arrived at Barbados the captain called the girl in and told her that she would have to leave the ship but that they would fly her back to London. She was devastated because she thought she'd lost her job but he tried to reassure her by saying it wasn't personal, it was for her own safety. The ship duly arrived in Miami where a trap had been set and a big smuggling operation was cleaned up.

Not long after I received a call from the girl's father, who was "something" in the Foreign Office. He told me in his best House and

Garden accent that he was going to sue both me and the shipping line because of the disgraceful treatment meted out to his daughter. It was outrageous as she had been absolutely beside herself at being shipped back to England. I waited until the bluster was over and told him he ought to be writing a letter of thanks to the captain for probably saving her life, instead of giving himself apoplexy and threatening to sue. He didn't have a clue about what had happened so I explained it all to him. I added for good measure that as she may well have been killed had she returned with the ship, because the gang may have thought it was her who shopped them, there was no way she could stay anywhere near Miami. He changed his tone almost immediately and thanked me profusely. I also told him that if she still wanted to work at sea then we had plenty of opportunities for her away from Miami and we did indeed take her back. I've often felt that the goings-on in an onboard salon would make good soap opera material.

Another girl, this time an American manageress on one of the Princess Line ships, was a problem in a different way. I started getting letters from the chief officer saying that there had been numerous passenger complaints about our service and that if it continued he would recommend that the contract be terminated. I was puzzled because I usually received any reports direct from the company and there had been no bad ones. I thought I'd better fly out to LA and see what the problem was. I soon noticed that the manageress appeared to be having an affair with this officer but I needed some evidence. I enlisted the help of one of the other girls by asking whether they had parties on board involving the manageress and other crew members. She confirmed that they had indeed had some great parties in the crew quarters. I asked her to take some photos of the next one because I was planning a little publication to illustrate how good staff/crew relations were on board. She fell for it and luckily one of her photos showed the manageress and the Chief Officer together, half-naked in a shower. I went straight to Princess saying I'd sacked my girl but it was up to them what they did with their man. Apparently she was after the concession herself and had used the Chief Officer to write letters trying to paint us in a bad light.

Another LA based story involving one of my British girls made the international press. Way back in the 80s there was a girl working in the gift shop of one the ships and she had fallen in love with an American passenger. This was an ever-present occupational hazard and it wasn't the first or last time this would happen although this one was the most complicated. They wanted to get married but the ship was based in LA and immigration wouldn't let her off the ship. Even if he'd married her on board she still wouldn't have been allowed off, she would have to go back to the UK and apply for a visa. Each time the ship arrived in LA, he would come to meet her on the quayside and she would be leaning over the rails gazing down at him. Well, the press picked this up and took a picture of just such a meeting. "Prisoner of Love" was the headline splashed over the papers the next day! My problem was that I needed to replace the girl but that immigration were watching her like hawks.

I went to LA with a replacement girl but also with a ticket for the original girl to fly back to London. I showed this to immigration and suggested they go with her to the airport and see her onto the plane. They agreed. Trouble was, the boyfriend didn't want her to go back but I managed to persuade him that this was the best way round it and he eventually went along with it. There was a happy ending: she got her visa and they got married, which is as it should have been.

The article in The Lady mentioned the ravages the salty sea air made on hair. It's true, the salt really takes a toll on hair and can leave it lank and lifeless which is no good if you're planning on getting dressed up for the captain's dinner. This later got me thinking and I wondered about the chances of marketing a range of products specifically for use at sea. Collagen was being used extensively in cosmetic surgery and I wondered whether it would work on hair. I had meetings with chemists and manufacturers and we came up with shampoo formulations that gave extra body to hair and also a conditioner that could be left in instead of being rinsed out. Our testing showed that it appeared to work well so we launched a range to use in the salons and to sell on board.

It sold OK until one of the directors of Royal Caribbean line came up with an idea. He suggested I call my products "Sir Anthony Kaye". I told him that I couldn't possibly give myself a title I hadn't been honoured with. It wasn't a problem in America, he said, as long as I registered it as a trade mark. When I checked it out I found that the name had been used before so I thought, "Bugger it, why not." From that moment on in America I traded as "Sir Anthony Kaye". The products were incredibly successful and sold like hot cakes on board.

The new name upset my competitors. I used to put on quite a flamboyant show at the annual Miami Sea Trades Convention and I had celebrated the name change by doing a big promotion. One of the opposition came over to me protesting that I couldn't call myself "Sir" and was calling me a fraud. I sent her away with a flea in her ear after pointing out to her the little trademark sign over the S of "Sir".

The name of course created some amusing incidences among our trans-Atlantic cousins. When I used to sell the products on board I would always give a bit of patter and the ladies lapped it up. "Your hair is lovely," I would say, "but it would really be enhanced by this product." And then show them the goods. Often I would get back "Are you who I think you are? Him?" they would say, pointing at my name on the bottle or can. "You know, you're such a clever lady. How did you guess?" The flattery always worked, just like on the market stall, and they'd buy loads of the stuff. Then they'd go off and tell their friends they'd actually met the real Sir Anthony Kaye. I didn't market them onshore at all but this word of mouth effect was unbelievable and I started a mail-order business, purely for America, on the back of it that eventually had a turnover of a couple of million dollars a year.

Regardless of the play acting on the ships where, to all intents and purposes, I was just the owner and the name on a can, the Americans, bless them, used to be (probably still are) very naïve and gullible when it comes to our class and title system. Playing along for fun is fine but one time I nearly landed myself in hot water.

I'd checked into a hotel and feeling tired because of my terribly aching back (this was before I had surgery on it), I just wanted to go to bed. I asked the receptionist if there was a doctor who could come out and see me. "Yes, Sir Kaye." She replied. I'm pretty certain my accent had thrown her and she assumed I was automatically entitled to a knighthood. I told her that if they were going to call me 'Sir' they couldn't call me "Sir Kaye", it would have to be either "Sir Anthony" or "Lord Kaye".

"We're very sorry your lordship, we'll get a doctor as quickly as possible!"

A few moments later there was a knock at the door. It was the doctor and he also addressed me as Sir Anthony. I asked him if he could prescribe me some powerful painkillers and he said he would get something special sent up as soon as possible. A few moments later the phone rang. It was the local television station: "Sir Anthony, we're sorry to trouble you but we have a talkshow on this evening and we'd like you to be our special guest." That's all I bloody need, I thought to myself. Now I was going to get done for fraud! I declined politely, saying my back was far too bad to venture out this evening.

"But we can bring our equipment to you and interview you in your room."

"Thank you for your kind offer but..."

Chapter 26
Presidents and Godmothers

I'm not a name dropper or dreadfully star-struck but I'll readily admit to having had the opportunity to meet some very well known people in some not quite so usual situations. It didn't happen very often though, celebrities don't often go cruising as being captive among a couple of thousand potential autograph hunters for a couple of weeks wouldn't necessarily be fun for them. The larger ships could attract well known cabaret acts for some sailings but generally the ships were celeb free.

The power of celebrity in America is very strong though and a couple of times I've been able to use this in business. One such occasion was in 1988. Royal Caribbean had just launched the Sovereign of the Seas, one of their first mega-ships. Tradition, in the US more so than in the rest of the world, dictates each ship should have a Godmother and the one chosen for the Sovereign was Rosalyn Carter, wife of ex-US President Jimmy Carter.

We obviously had a presence on board with the salon but we also had a health and fitness centre, fitted out with the latest computerised machinery. When I heard that the Carters would be coming on board I had some red, white and blue striped clothing made up for them and they loved it! Jimmy Carter was a well-known fitness enthusiast so I asked him if he would mind posing on some the rowing machines and other machinery for some photos. To my delight he agreed and he also agreed when I asked permission to use the pictures of him in Bally's (the manufacturer) brochure. At the end of the cruise I called Bally and asked them if they'd be interested in some real publicity for their new equipment. They told me it would have to be someone big for them to be interested.

"What about the ex-President of the United States?" I suggested.

"Jimmy Carter?"

"I've got pictures of Jimmy Carter on the machines and what's more, I've also got a signed release. If you don't believe me, come and have a look." Which they did, flying over from their base in California. They were beside themselves when they saw the pictures and they asked me how much I wanted for them. I got 50% back on the price of the equipment I'd just bought from them for a small fortune, which I thought was a pretty good deal!

I also have a letter from the Carters thanking me for introducing them to aromatherapy while they were on board. In fact, Jimmy was so taken with it he asked if we could train up his maid as a practitioner. I still have pictures of them both, kitted out in my stars and stripes kit!

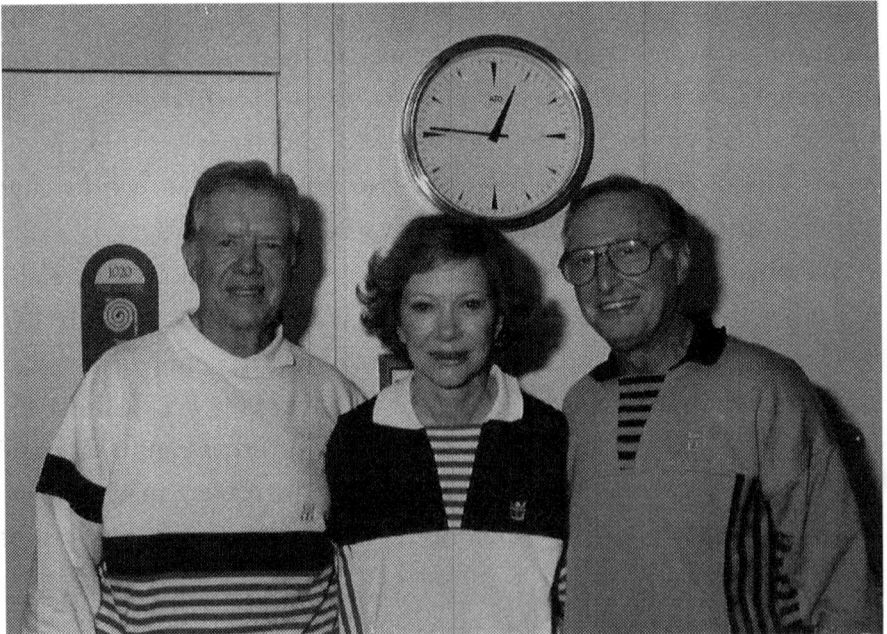

Jimmy and Rosalyn Carter

I've been lucky enough to witness many other launchings and naming ceremonies but one that sticks in the memory involved Margaret Thatcher, who named the Regal Princess in 1991 in New York. No expense had been spared as the Band of the Coldstream Guards struck up "There is Nothing Like a Dame" as she ascended the podium. There were some amazing scenes as the crowd went wild, shouting "We want Maggie for President!" On board, following the ceremony she was presented with a silver plate by P & O and Fincantieri, the shipyard, gave her an exquisite gold bracelet. That moment the Iron Lady's guard dropped and she turned into a woman, simpering like a young girl saying how beautiful it was. It was a sight I'm sure not many people had seen before.

Princess Diana on the other hand reacted in a quite down-to-earth fashion after naming the Royal Princess at Southampton in 1984. She came on board to look around, visited the salon and exclaimed, "Oh my God! Your manicures are very expensive!" I couldn't think of a reply to that!

Besides the Godmother tradition, there was one other that could have some quite unusual outcomes. Many of the mega-ships were built at the Finnish shipyards. In Finland it's traditional that on a ship's completion the workers and their families are invited on board where drinks and food are served. The first time I arrived at one of these ceremonies I saw a fleet of ambulances lined up on the quayside and I thought something dreadful had happened until I was told the truth. Apparently, the other, rather less formal, part of the tradition was for the guys to drink so much vodka as to be nigh on incapable. This meant that when the party was over and they left the warmth of the ship, the effect of the icy sub-zero air on them would knock them out by the time they'd reached the bottom of the gangway. The ambulances were there to collect the inevitable casualties. I was on the Song of America after one such party and we set off straight away for Oslo the moment the party finished. I was sitting with some of the executives having a drink in the lounge when suddenly, at the other end of the room, a man got up from between the tables, shouted "Hey, you!" and fell down again. He kept popping up all over the room, shouting the same thing and collapsing – obviously someone the ambulances had forgotten!

For my salons I used the services of a great designer called John Picken. When I got the contracts for the Royal Caribbean Sovereign class ships I asked John if he wanted to join the company. He said he would but that he would need to bring in a colleague to help with the workload. I then thought that it would be a good idea to form a separate design company so, as John's design partner was called Stephen Frasier, in 1989 we formed Stephenjohn Design, with John as managing director. We were awarded the contract to design the spa on the Norway, the largest passenger liner then afloat (but as I write this, currently grounded off a beach in India with her fate as yet undecided) and it was a triumph. The Roman Spa, as it was named, was only the second complete self-contained spa area built on any ship, mainly because the Norway was one of the few around that had enough available space to accommodate all the equipment and facilities in one place. It attracted a lot of interest at the Miami spa convention held just after we finished it, not least because I convinced Norwegian America Line to invite all the delegates onto the ship to see the spa. The upshot of that was that spas became part of the cruising experience and not just a sideshow hidden away in the bowels of the ship.

Everybody is due 15 minutes of fame, according to Andy Warhol, and I would be no exception to this considering that the American measure of fame is a TV appearance. The quiz show "Wheel of Fortune" is huge in the US and its hostess, Vanna White is one of the nation's darlings. In 1994 they were to record an edition of the show from on board the SS Norway. I spoke to the producer, Nancy Jones, and suggested they could feature the Roman Spa and that we could offer a prize. She loved the spa and thought the idea was great. So did I: free advertising worth millions on one of the country's biggest TV shows? You can't buy luck like that! Nancy told me that I would have to write 10 seconds of copy for the announcer. I tried and tried but I just couldn't get it down past 14 seconds and I gave it to her expecting her to cut it. "Don't worry," she said, "number one, you don't know how fast my announcer can talk and two, you can have a couple of seconds extra anyway."

Dick Carson, the director (and brother of Johnny Carson the US talk show legend) came over to me and asked me what on earth I'd done to Nancy: "She never gives two seconds to anyone!"

Dick also said that he wanted me to film with Vanna White and asked me whether I'd ever worked in front of camera before. I told him I hadn't but he told me not to worry about it and to just relax. I got into a tracksuit, suitable attire for a health and fitness club, and was introduced to Vanna. I had to apologise to her. "Forgive me saying this but everybody's telling me that I'm going to be filming with Vanna White and I'm asking "Vanna who? I'm sorry but I've never heard of you! I suppose I ought to be embarrassed because everybody here knows you. I'm just a miserable Englishman!" At which she roared with laughter. Dick Carson came over and told me I needn't worry about relaxing in front of camera, I was doing great already! The show was a success and we had a lot of interest as a result and Stephenjohn Design Ltd went on to become the world leaders in spa design. In the picture on the back cover of this book I'm actually standing in front of a poster of the Roman Spa taken during the recording of 'Wheel of Fortune'. As you can also see, I've still got some Sir Anthony Kaye samples left!

-oo0oo-

I've loved meeting people from all walks of life and I've made many many friends over the years. I've also been lucky enough to meet a few show-business personalities "off-guard" so to speak. Many years ago a friend of my first wife had a brother who was an actor, Glynn

Edwards was his name. He's probably best known as Dave, the barman from "Minder" the television series starring George Cole and Dennis Waterman. Glynn invited us to a party at his house and one of the other guests was the wonderful Roy Kinnear. Until his tragic death from the injuries he received falling off a horse while filming "the Return of the Musketeers" in 1988, Roy was one of our best and most familiar comic actors. He and his wife Carmel subsequently became very great friends and he was an automatic guest at any party, where his ebullience would always lighten the proceedings. Ironically, in the late 70s Roy played a character in a TV sitcom called "No Appointment Necessary" by the name of Alf Butler; Alf was a greengrocer who also ran a hairdressing salon.

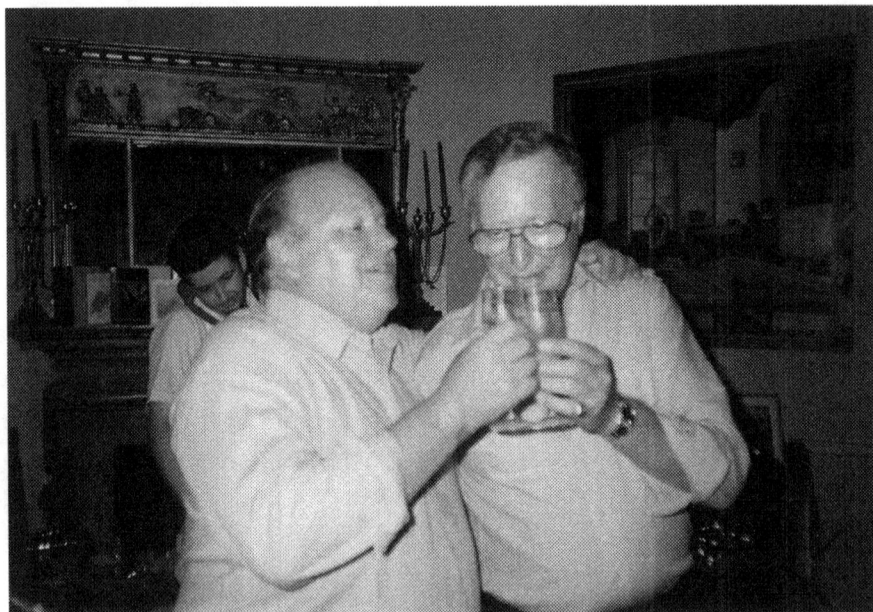

One of my best friends, the late Roy Kinnear, being the life and soul, as ever

I think laughter is so important, I see so many people without a sense of humour and wonder how on earth they can get through the day. Roy could be the life and soul of the party but he never imposed and he wore his celebrity lightly. My kind of person and I miss him a great deal.

I once invited Roy and another good friend, broadcaster Susie Barnes, to a dinner I'd arranged with some P & O directors because I thought it would make a change from the normal stuffy business meeting. Besides, I'd been trying to get in with P & O for ages with no luck so decided a different approach was needed. Before we started I made it clear that nobody was to be caught discussing business or contracts at all otherwise I'd ask them to leave; it was to be a purely social occasion. Roy was on top form and it was a great evening. Eventually the P & O crowd had to leave around 1am in order to head back to Southampton. On the way out one of them asked me why I'd not allowed business talk as they were convinced I'd held the dinner to play for contracts. I replied, "I told you, no business. But tomorrow I'll be knocking on your door asking "how's about a contract?" Not because of the dinner though but because I know we can do it better than anybody else." They looked at me and felt convinced.

Another good friend was ex-Olympic sprinter and captain of Britain's 1968 Olympic team, Ron Jones. Ron had a position at Queen's Park Rangers football club and would often invite Alexis and me to home games at their Loftus Road ground. His guests would all congregate in his office before and after the game for a drink. We were a pretty mixed bunch, too. Rock drummer Phil Collins, Radio 1 DJ David "Kid" Jensen, Susie Barnes and Linda, Ron's girlfriend were frequent guests. For Alexis' 7th birthday Ron had the great idea of kitting him out in a replica kit and leading the team out as the club mascot. This hadn't been done before as far as we knew and his first game was against Manchester United. He was featured in the match programme and some magazine articles and the game was also televised. The idea caught on and it's rare today to see a team without a child realising his or her dream and leading their heroes out. He was also given the match ball signed by both teams and the great Stan

Bowles gave him his No 9 shirt, also signed. Sadly, his allegiance changed after my brother started taking him to see Spurs when QPR were playing away!

Somebody else I came to know very well was the entertainer Frankie Vaughan. It was a curious meeting though as our friendship was more or less engineered! In the early 80s, Frank took a Royal Caribbean cruise. A good friend of mine, Bob Perez, who was RCCL's shore side executive, told Frank that he ought to meet me because we had a lot in common. A while later, and completely out of the blue, I got a call from Frank telling me what a good time he'd had on board and what Bob had told him about me. He was doing a charity show at the London Palladium and invited me and a guest to meet him afterwards.

The show overran and as he was tired Frank went home early, sending us an apology and also saying that he'd contact me. He was as good as his word and phoned me that week to invite me over to his home in Totteridge for dinner. On the way over I started to wonder why I was going. We appeared to have nothing in common and I was getting cold feet. Even as he welcomed me and served drinks I was still a bit bothered by what we'd find to talk about.

I needn't have worried as we started to talk about musicians and in doing so found out that we had a mutual friend in Bert Weedon, which broke the ice. When the subject got on to my wrestling promoting days all the barriers came down and we got on famously. He took me to his favourite Indian restaurant and it was a delicious meal but I was amazed to see him tuck into his favourite dish, which just happened to be the hottest one on the menu. From that day until the sad one in 1999 when he passed away, we were great friends and Stella, his wife, remains so to this day.

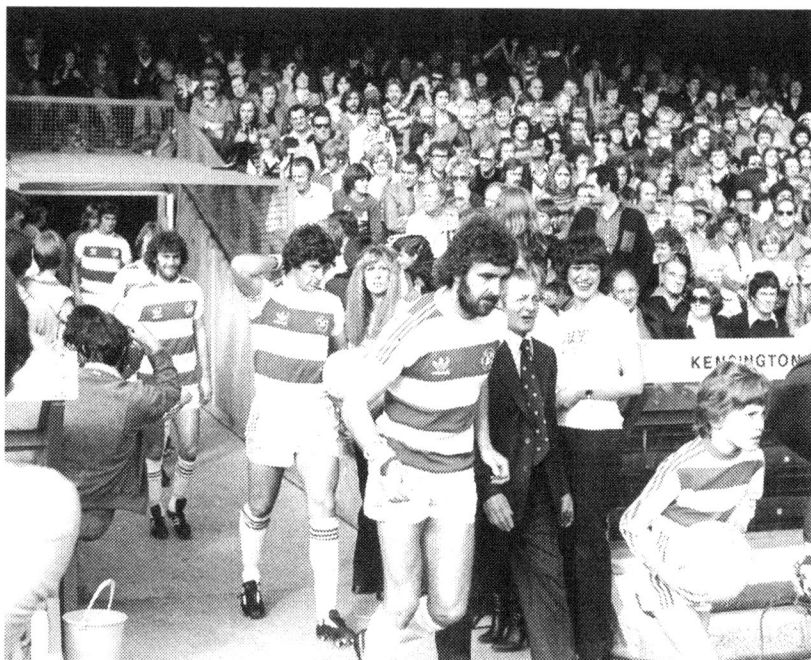

Alexis Leading QPR out in 1978

Chapter 27
Miami Times

Because the company offices were in Miami and I was spending so much time in America, I bought a house on Miami's Fisher Island. Although I lived there much of the time, I never took American citizenship, in fact I hung resolutely on to my British accent even vowing to teach the locals proper English! People used to ask me how I felt now that I was surrounded by the rich and famous but I used to reply that I didn't feel any different because I still liked nothing better than to sit down with a cup of tea and a bacon sandwich. Seeing people change with success can be intensely annoying although I have to say that once your success is acknowledged by your peers, it can be very useful in opening doors in business.

One particular success I had was in applying for a coveted green card. This allowed me to avoid immigration when travelling in and out of the country, which could be a real pain when you consider the number of vessels we operated on that went outside US territorial waters. Luckily I was fortunate enough to get to know the heads of customs over the years and was able to arrange on-board clearances. The head of customs at Miami alternated between the docks and the airport and when I arrived on a plane he would arrange for me to go through crew immigration, meeting me at the end of the airbridge and escorting me through. One time I came off with a holdall, which he offered to carry for me. I said it could be full of dope for all he knew. "If it is," he replied, "we're partners."

Another time I'd bought a present back for a girlfriend in Miami from the American duty free island of St Thomas in the US Virgin Islands. I asked the chief of customs whether I could do the clearance on board. He said it was OK but asked what I had to declare. When I told him he just waved it aside saying it was nothing and not to worry. I then gave him a $10 tip to pass on to the porters, who were helping me to get my stuff unloaded. He immediately held it up and said loudly, "I want you all to make a note of this: bribery!" We had such an easy relationship with everybody.

In the late 80s some friends of mine in Miami got me talking about my time in the music business and especially my time with George Shearing. One day they called me up and told me they had a big surprise for me: George was playing Miami and they had tickets. We went and it was a great concert and featured George playing alongside other great pianists, Marian McPartland being one of them. After the show my friends suggested that as I had told them so much about George, why didn't I go down to the dressing room and see him? "Listen," I said. "It's been 40 years since I worked with George and he's been blind since birth, it'll be bloody difficult for me to go down there, introduce myself and expect him to remember." My friends gave me the kind of looks that suggested they weren't going to believe my original stories anymore. Well, we got down to the lobby only to be met with the sight of George sitting at a table with Marian, autographing his latest record. My friends told me I could hardly make excuses now so reluctantly I joined the end of the queue of people paying $10 for the record then getting it signed.

As we got nearer I was wondering how to introduce myself. Was there anything I could think of to jog his memory as obviously he couldn't see me? When I finally got to the end of the line I said to him, "George, it's Tony Kaye. I still feel sick every time I think of you eating pickles and porridge in Lyons Corner House in Coventry Street!" George stopped dead in his tracks, turned his head up towards me and said, "Tony Kaye? What are you doing here?" And off we went reminiscing. But to cap it all, Marian then came up and started on me, "For crying out loud! Don't you remember me? We played together too!" Unfortunately I couldn't but nevertheless my friends were really impressed. There was a restaurant locally that had live jazz playing so we all went off and had dinner and thankfully my friends never queried my stories again!

One of my girls, a beautician, said she was going to leave because she was marrying the maître d' of the ship she was on and they were going to start up a business in Texas. I told her I was very sorry to see her go because I'd plans for her but I wished her well. I heard later that she'd gone to work in a local salon and that he was working in a restaurant so maybe their plans hadn't worked out.

A couple of years later my receptionist put a call through to me saying it was from an ex-staff member. I didn't recognise the name but it turned out to be the same girl, now married. She said she was in Miami and would like to see me. When we met later that afternoon she said that they had both left their jobs and had opened their own restaurant. It had been very successful so they'd opened another, then another and so on until they had a chain. She was in Miami because they had a new one on Bayside and she was asking if I would officially open it for them. She told me that I was the nicest person she'd worked for and that she wanted me to share in her success. That is what I call a reward.

Another restaurant many of the shipping executives and I used to visit in Miami for lunch was also often frequented by a senior judge and one day we were in there at the same time as he was. Pandemonium broke loose as the place was surrounded by police and FBI, who arrested the judge. Allegedly he had been taking backhanders off the mob and they'd found $50,000 in the boot of his car.

Incidentally, Pietro Venezia, the owner of the restaurant and an ex-waiter from one of the Royal Viking Line ships was also in trouble. He hadn't paid his tax returns so the IRS closed his bank accounts down meaning he couldn't pay his bills or his staff. Venezia was understandably angry and unfortunately he also knew where the tax inspector lived. On Christmas Eve 1993 he got into his car, drove out to the tax inspector's home and waited for him to arrive. When he did,

Venezia pulled out a gun and shot him dead. Then he calmly got into his car, drove to the airport and flew to Rome. He was put on trial in Italy but the judge ruled that he couldn't be extradited back to Florida because he would face the death penalty.

I've always loved sport. As an Englishman, obviously cricket and football but my big love is tennis. Back home in England during Wimbledon fortnight I used to hold tennis barbecue parties at my house in Swiss Cottage. I'd invite many names from the world of tennis and other sports as well as my own close friends. I got quite involved with tennis for many years, making many friends along the way. In the late 80s I discovered the Alpha Massage System in America. This was a revolutionary new system that involved climbing inside what looked like a mini spaceship and getting your back massaged in an atmosphere of ionised air with your favourite music playing if you wanted. They were very relaxing and very therapeutic.

I thought that tennis pros could benefit from these so I enlisted the help of my friend Jim Westhall, the then promoter of the New Haven, Connecticut tournament, one of the run-up tournaments to the US Open. We installed one of the machines there and it generated huge TV interest. Then I put them in the Lipton tournament at Key Biscayne and from there into the Nick Bollettieri Tennis Academy. The climax came when I managed to get them into Wimbledon. It was certainly a long way from hairstyling! When I eventually disposed of my companies I closed this part down as it involved many personal friendships and contacts I didn't want to lose under a new owner.

-ooOoo-

In 1991 I began to notice that my voice wasn't carrying and that I was always needing to clear my throat. I went to see a doctor friend who lived near me on Fisher Island and he in turn sent me to an ear, nose and throat man. He had a look and said I had a growth on a vocal chord and that he could zap it off with a laser and after a week without speaking I'd be fine. Sometimes we trust what our bodies are telling us more than what we hear from the doctors and my body was telling me that what I was hearing from this man wasn't right. I spoke to another friend, this time a theatre nurse. They tend to know all the reputations and rumours as far as doctors go and she recommended I go and see another specialist. I did and after a much more extensive examination he told me that it wasn't just a simple growth, it went the whole length of the vocal chord and that laser treatment wouldn't clear it, I'd need radiation treatment.

Now I was totally perplexed and sought a third opinion. I went back to my nurse friend and she said that despite it being a human zoo, the Jackson Memorial Hospital was the place to go. There they put a camera down my throat and it showed that it looked like Mt Vesuvius around my larynx. According to the specialist there was a 95% certainty that it was malignant. A biopsy proved that it was indeed cancerous and that radiation therapy would be the only course of action that would leave my vocal chords relatively undamaged. I started treatment for cancer of the larynx immediately, treatment that would ultimately entail 5 days of therapy a week over two and a half months - but at least I didn't have to undergo invasive surgery.

Usually they mark you with a small tattoo upon which the radiation beam is focused. With me they made me a fibreglass mask and marked that instead. There were side effects: my throat swelled up and it was difficult to swallow. They said I'd have to give up eating solids about halfway through the treatment as well but I didn't. I'm not very good when it comes to obeying doctor's orders and I carried on working and also playing tennis but all the specialists agreed that it was this positive attitude that helped me overcome the cancer so well. The same positive attitude I'd used throughout my working life.

I was given the all clear in 1996, 5 years after treatment finished. Just prior to writing this I visited my specialist again because recently I've found my voice starts to deteriorate quickly when I'm speaking. He had a look but said I had nothing to worry about, there was no chance of the cancer re-occurring. Unfortunately it was just that I was getting old and wearing out and with the best will in the world, there wasn't much he could do about that. Thanks, doc!

Chapter 28
For Sale

At the Miami Sea Trades Convention in 1993 I put on a lavish show to celebrate the 30th anniversary of Coiffeur Transocean. There was much talk about taking the company forward into the 21st century. The problem was I was now beginning to get a bit tired of being woken up at all hours with problems from China or California so I eventually asked Alexis if he wanted to join the company. If he didn't want to, I'd sell. He didn't and Steiners got word of this and made me an offer I would have had trouble refusing. The attraction for any buyer was the inherent potential in a captive market; open a salon in the High Street and you've got to fight all the other salons for a small slice of the pie. Open a salon on a cruise ship and the whole pie is yours if you want it. Guaranteed.

I sold the lot apart from the name, design company and the massage machine business. Steiners had their own well-known name so they didn't need mine plus I think they were really after my database from the mail-order business. That's fair enough but whether they were ever able to capitalise on this, I don't know as I'm certain my US customers were really only interested in buying the Sir Anthony Kaye range. I'm sure they thought they knew what they were doing.

The majority of my staff transferred over but I would often hear back from them that it wasn't the same. Many were in tears when the sale was announced. Even those who had come to CT from the competitors said that although the conditions were similar, the atmosphere was totally different, much more like a family. One of my vice-presidents, Elaine Fenard, originally from Wales, came to me and told me she could never work for the new company, saying I'd been like a father to her and that I'd taught her everything. I said I was very touched but that it was her future and she had to think of that. She stayed for a year then joined the Starwood Hotels group where she was in charge of their spa operations. She's now recognised as one of the leading authorities in the spa industry. One or two of my executives also did very well from the sale and as I write, Leonard Fluxman, my old VP of Finance is the President and CEO of Steiner Leisure.

I gave the rest of my shares in Stephenjohn Design to John Picken and the company is going from strength to strength, designing spas and salons on virtually every newbuilding ship and for many land-based concerns such as hotels. The fact that I've been able to give starts to people such John fills me with joy. All being said, I was happy to sell up because once the shipping companies became public companies, all they became interested in was the bottom line. Everyone but the customer was getting squeezed for more and more and it was getting very difficult to turn a profit. If a company can't make a profit, everyone in it suffers.

Part of the deal was that neither I nor Alexis was allowed to start up again in the same business as a competitor for a period of five or six years after the sale. To ensure the take-over ran smoothly, Steiners also employed me as a consultant for two years following the sale. Many of the shipping companies CT were contracted to weren't happy with the sale and my presence helped to placate their fears. However it was a situation that presented its own set of unusual problems because although I was on the payroll, I'm not sure my new employers realised what an asset I could be to them.

One occasion was like a scene from a comedy film. Royal Caribbean held a luncheon on board a ship after its naming ceremony and because I was friends with the senior executives they invited me to join them at the top table. Sitting next to me was another old acquaintance, a Greek ship owner. We were having a laugh and a joke because I was ribbing him about the "bloody old banger" he'd bought, suggesting that he turn it into a "Love Boat" for singles to travel on. The dining room was several stories high and we were on the lowest one. My new boss was sat a story higher up but had been watching me intently and, curious to know what I'd been discussing, had been phoning another one of his employees sat at a table nearer to us. When he confronted me later I told him that we had actually been discussing him and calling him the biggest shit in the world. He had no sense of humour at all so I had to remind him that I'd been in the business for over 30 years and knew everybody worth knowing. If I hadn't known everybody after all this time, I certainly wouldn't be his consultant now as he wouldn't now own the company I'd built up on the strength of some of those contacts. He then told me that he'd been trying to get an appointment with the Greek for ages but had been repeatedly ignored. "Why didn't you ask me then? I can do it."

The only time I was tempted to go back into business was a few years ago after one of my tennis/barbecue parties that I used to hold at my old home in Swiss Cottage. The cheap flights pioneer Sir Freddie Laker's wife was a guest (I had known them both from Fisher Island as they were neighbours) and she said that Freddie was coming out of retirement to start a new airline venture. I thought to myself that maybe it wasn't too late to have another go at something but then thought of all the failures one may have to go through before success is realised. Not for me, though. At the age I sold up, I didn't think I had enough years left to spend waiting for success to come around again. Maybe I should have taken a lead from another of my good friends from Miami, Gardner Mulloy, the tennis champion. He's still playing tennis well in his 90s!

Coiffeur Transocean was like a family in many ways. I had tried to remain approachable even though I was the owner. As I've mentioned time and again, I hate pretence in any walk of life – after all, deep down I'm still that same East End market trader who started out selling books – and I've always tried to stay grounded. I also firmly believe in the old adage that you should be nice to people on the way up, because you never know when you'll need them on the way down. When I used to travel down to Southampton from London, if any of the staff were with me they were always amazed when I used to pull in at a transport café for a cup of tea and a full English breakfast. "How can you do that?" they used to ask me. "Simple," I'd reply, "I order eggs, bacon, beans and a fried slice!" Why on earth should I have forgotten my roots just because I've been successful?

The sale of the company meant I was liable for a huge amount of tax so I asked my tax lawyer for some ideas on how I could minimise it. One option was to make myself a resident of Grand Cayman for a year but in order to 'qualify' I would have to embrace an equivalent lifestyle with a similar size house to what I had in the US. As I've said before, I'm a city person and the thought of being marooned on Grand Cayman for a year was terrible; I'd feel like Napoleon exiled on St Helena. Another option was that if I was heading back to Europe anyway, why not go to Monaco, which is a well-known tax haven. I'd still be liable for some tax under this arrangement but not all of it, because of the way in which the money from the sale was being paid to me. It seemed to me to be a bigger draw than Grand Cayman, so I agreed and sold my Miami home in 1996.

Before I went I made out the biggest cheque I'd ever written, paying what I owed to the IRS. I thought it was horrendous and I was shaking. I'd got to give all this money away that I'd spent all my life working for, on top of all the tax that I'd already paid, just because I'd sold the company. I bit the bullet, ruminating on the fact that I wouldn't have been in that situation had I not been in America anyway.

I also had to give up my Green Card and that involved coming back to London to the US Embassy, as that was where it had been issued. That episode was amusing in itself as there were crowds of people all queuing up there to apply for green cards and visas. A guy came along the line directing people to the right place. When he got to me he asked me what I wanted and I said I wanted to surrender my green card. I don't think those surrounding me could believe what they were hearing: who on earth was this crazy man giving up the holy grail of a US green card?

Getting in to Monaco wasn't easy either. First I needed to get a visa from the French Embassy. Odd, considering one only usually needs a passport to travel to France. Then I had to have a medical with their doctors and I also had to provide all my personal documents such as bank statements, divorce proof, police record etc to satisfy the authorities that I wasn't going to be a liability to the tiny principality. Finally I had to open a bank account and then wait two weeks for my application to be approved. During that time I went to Monaco to look for somewhere to live. The very final act after approval was to register for a resident's permit with the police.

The following January I returned to the UK to look for a home in London as I felt that one day in the future I would return for good. I looked at several but the one I wanted and felt most comfortable in needed extensive work done on it. I hired my old design company to rebuild the interior and that was finished by September 1997, when The Times did their feature.

I was in Monaco for several years but I got tired with it in the end. I don't speak a lot of French and there really wasn't a lot for me to do there, it's very small after all. I occasionally went to the opera and ballet, otherwise I was lucky if there was one English language film a week I could enjoy. The others were all dubbed and I hate watching Dustin Hoffman with a French actor's voice.

One thing annoyed me above all else and that was the name-dropping and one-upmanship among all the ex-pats; that snobbery thing that I hate appearing again. Bugger it, I thought, I really can't put up with this any longer, I'll go back to England. I did in late 2003 and I've never regretted it. Neither did the Inland Revenue who welcomed me back with wide-open arms!

I had rented my flat in Monaco and I needed to get rid of it as there was still time on the lease. I went back to the estate agent in Monaco to instruct them to organise a new tenant but he was such a snob he could barely bring himself to look at me.

I returned to London but went back to Monaco a couple of weeks later. My first thought was to go and see this bastard of an estate agent and tell him where to get off. I went into his office and he was a changed man, fawning all over me, offering me coffee and a seat. He told me he'd just been showing somebody round my flat and he'd seen photographs of me meeting a few celebrities and this seemed to excite him no end. "I didn't know you were friends with President Carter and Princess Margarethe of Sweden" he crawled. I looked at him and stopped him in his tracks. "Don't go any further. Is this the only way I can get decent treatment from you? Because you've seen photographs of me meeting them you think I actually know these people? I'll tell you what you can do, you can go and see a taxidermist, I'm taking my business elsewhere!" And with that, I stormed out.

I've also never been comfortable talking about money. That all started back when I was working in the markets. If I'd made a lot of sales I used to empty my pockets and count the money and that in turn made my father shout at me to never count money outside because you never want to show everyone how much you're making. The distaste I subsequently felt has spread to any kind of bragging: Monaco, a town built entirely on status through wealth, certainly wasn't the place for me.

Chapter 29
And Finally...

All the experiences I had during my life were ultimately helpful to me in the hairdressing and salon business afloat. It doesn't matter what one does, an experience of any kind always leaves a mark, each one something to be learned from.

The people though, they are the great unsung teachers. I was so lucky to have worked in New York with Caruso and Eddie Senz and meeting all those wonderful people with whom I became friends, not because I forced myself on them but because they enjoyed what I was doing with their hair.

Making friends is still one of my greatest pleasures and I'm fortunate in that I'm able to get on with people. Several years ago I went on a round the world tour deliberately going to places I've never visited before. I went alone and without an itinerary and this surprised a lot of people I met. It's the way I am and it's so much more fun that way as one never knows what or who is around the next corner. In every country I visited on that tour I made friends. A Malaysian couple, on honeymoon in Australia when I first met them, even flew to Britain to meet up with me and I take actions like that as a great compliment. I'm often the last person to leave a restaurant because I end up having drinks with the manager or chef.

People are fun to be around. Getting people to open up and have a laugh is a challenge to me and it's the same philosophy that sustained me during my business career. After all, it's easier to make contracts and work with people you like and can trust, even if sometimes I've had to employ some of that old streetwise market trader nous on the way.

Ironically, considering the number I've been on, I don't like the close confines of a ship and I was always happy to get off. I'm very much a big city person and love the choice of theatres, concerts and restaurants one gets in cities. Even those three and half wonderful months in Montego Bay made me feel strangely claustrophobic as every time I went outside I felt I could stretch out my arms and touch each side of the island. Every time I boarded the plane for New York, I breathed a sigh of relief that soon I would be back among people and making new friends.

I don't regret anything. Sometimes I wonder what may have happened had I kept on with the wrestling promotions or stayed in music. Would I have been as happy? Probably not in the long run because that combination of itchy feet and the nagging feeling eating away at you all the time, convincing you that what you're doing is only a stepping stone, always proved too much and I had to move on. It was a great journey.

-ooOoo-

To all the gentlemen and villains I've had either the good or misfortune to meet in this wonderful life I've led: you've all left your marks. I'm a mixture of you all and I thank you for making it all possible.